CHECK POINT INHIBITORS

A NEW CLASS OF DRUGS FOR CANCER TREATMENT

A book in the Modern Medicine Series

Kerry Atkinson MD DTM&H FRACP FRCP

About this book

The information describing check point inhibitors is taken from the USA Food and Drug Administration's Prescribing Highlights and the FDA's Full Prescribing Information for each drug. Both these documents are in the public domain.

All other text was written by the author. Some text written by the author occurs within the FDA descriptions: in this case, the text by the author is placed in *italics* and the section is placed in (parentheses).

All images used in this book are in the public domain and the reason for their being in the public domain is detailed next to each respective image.

Acknowledgements

I would like to acknowledge the help that I received from Jim Severino in designing the covers for this book and for uploading it for me to Kindle Direct Publishing.

Key words: immune check point inhibitors; cancer medicine; new drugs for cancer; improvements in cancer treatment; monoclonal antibodies; combination therapy for cancer

Other books by Kerry Atkinson

Medical books

1. Graft-versus-Host Disease. Editors, S Burakoff, H J Deeg, J Ferrara, K Atkinson. Marcel Dekker Inc, New York, 1990.
2. Clinical Bone Marrow Transplantation. First edition. Editor, K Atkinson. Cambridge University Press, Cambridge UK, 1994.
3. The BMT Data Book: A Manual for Bone Marrow and Blood Stem Cell Transplantation. K. Atkinson, Cambridge University Press, Cambridge UK, 1998.
4. Clinical Bone Marrow and Blood Stem Cell Transplantation. Second Edition. Editor, K. Atkinson. Cambridge University Press, Cambridge UK, 2000.
5. Clinical Bone Marrow and Blood Stem Cell Transplantation. Third Edition. Eds, K. Atkinson, R Champlin, J Ritz, M Brenner, P Ljungman and W Fibbe. Cambridge University Press, Cambridge UK, 2004.
6. The BMT Data Book. Second edition. R Munker, HM Lazarus and K. Atkinson, Cambridge University Press, Cambridge UK, 2009.
7. The BMT Data Book: Including Cellular Therapy. Third edition. R Munker, C Hildebrandt, HM Lazarus and K. Atkinson, Cambridge University Press, Cambridge UK. 2013.
8. Hematopoietic Cell Transplants: Concepts, Controversies and Future Directions. Eds HM Lazarus, RP Gale, A Keating, A Bacigalupo, R Munker, K Atkinson, A Syed. Cambridge University Press, Cambridge, UK. 2017.
9. The Biology and Therapeutic Application of Mesenchymal Cells. Ed. K Atkinson. Wiley/Blackwell. 2017
10. Revolutionizing Tropical Medicine. Eds. K Atkinson and D Mabey. Wiley/Blackwell Publishers Inc. 2019.
11. Asthma: Targeted Biological Treatments 2020. Kindle Direct Publishing, 2020. e-book and paperback
12. Atopic Dermatitis: Targeted Biological Treatments 2020. Kindle Direct Publishing, 2020. e-book and paperback
13. Psoriasis: Targeted Biological Treatments 2020. Kindle Direct Publishing, 2020. e-book and paperback
14. Crohn's disease and ulcerative colitis: Targeted Biological Treatments 2020. Kindle Direct Publishing, 2020. e-book and paperback

15. Rheumatoid arthritis, Juvenile Idiopathic Arthritis, Ankylosing spondylitis, Psoriatic Arthritis and Gout: Targeted Biological Treatments 2020. Kindle Direct Publishing, 2020. e-book and paperback
16. Small Cell Lung Cancer: Targeted Biological Treatments 2020. Kindle Direct Publishing, 2020. e-book and paperback
17. Chronic Myeloid Leukemia: Targeted Biological Treatments 2020. Kindle Direct Publishing, 2020. e-book and paperback
18. Melanoma: Targeted Biological Treatments 2020, Kindle Direct Publishing 2020. e-book and paperback
19. Dementia - A Caregiver's Guide. Kindle Direct Publishing 2020. e-book
20. Breast Cancer: Targeted Biological Treatments 2021. Kindle Direct Publishing 2021. e-book and paperback
21. Non-melanoma Skin Cancers: Targeted Biological and Specifically Designed Therapeutic agents. 2022. Kindle Direct Publishing 2021. e-book and paperback
22. Hodgkin Lymphoma: Targeted Biological Treatments. 2022. Kindle Direct Publishing 2022. e-book and paperback
23. Chimeric Antigen Receptor (CAR) T Cells: The second Revolution in Cellular Therapy. 2022. Kindle Direct Publishing 2022. e-book and paperback
24. Acute lymphoblastic leukemia: targeted immune therapeutic agents. Kindle Direct Publishing 2023. e-book and paperback
25. Artificial Intelligence and Medicine. A book in the Modern Medicine series. Kindle Direct Publishing 2024. e-book and paperback

Natural history/conservation books

26. Bird facts for everyone. K Atkinson. Outskirts Press Inc., Denver, USA. 2014
27. Birds, Birds, Birds. Kindle Direct Publishing 2020. e-book and paperback
28. A Field Guide to the Wild Habitats of Sydney Australia. Kindle Direct Publishing 2021. e-book and paperback
29. Conserving New Zealand's Endangered Species. Kindle Direct Publishing 2021. e-book and paperback
30. Conserving Australia's Endangered Species. Kindle Direct Publishing 2021. e-book and paperback

31. Nature's Wonders: Britain and Ireland. Kindle Direct Publishing 2021. e-book and paperback.
32. Nature's Wonders: Spain and Bulgaria. Kindle Direct Publishing 2022. e-book and paperback.
33. Nature's Wonders: France's Camargue, the Swiss National Park and Portugal. Kindle Direct Publishing 2022. e-book and paperback.
34. Nature's Wonders: Cuba. Kindle Direct Publishing 2022. e-book and paperback.
35. Nature's Wonders: Japan in Winter Kindle Direct Publishing 2022. e-book and paperback.
36. Nature's Wonders: India. Kindle Direct Publishing 2022. e-book and paperback.
37. Nature's Wonders: Tanzania. Kindle Direct Publishing 2022. e-book and paperback.
38. The Silk Road: Uzbekistan and Kazakhstan – A Book in the Nature's Wonders Series. 2022. Kindle Direct Publishing 2022. e-book and paperback.
39. Madagascar – Land of Lemurs and Chameleons: a book in the Nature's Wonders series 2023. Kindle Direct Publishing 2022. e-book and paperback.
40. South Africa - Kalahari to the Cape - a book in the Nature's Wonders series. Kindle Direct Publishing 2022. e-book and paperback
41. Nature's Wonders – Finland - land of owls and lakes. Kindle Direct Publishing 2023. e-book and paperback
42. Nature's Wonders – Ethiopia. Kindle Direct Publishing 2023. e-book and paperback
43. Nature's Wonders – Kakadu National Park and Central Australia. Kindle Direct Publishing 2023. e-book and paperback
44. Nature's Wonders – Lord Howe Island, Australia. Kindle Direct Publishing 2023. e-book and paperback
45. Norway above the Arctic Circle in March. A book in the Nature's Wonders series. Kindle Direct Publishing 2024. e-book and paperback
46. The Inside Passage and the Pribilof Islands. A book in the Nature's Wonders series. Kindle Direct Publishing 2024. e-book and paperback
47. Orca! A book in the Nature's Wonders series. Kindle Direct Publishing 2024. e-book

Other books

48. Paintings by Kerry Atkinson 2019 – 2021. Kindle Direct Publishing 2021. e-book and paperback.
49. Ferrari Road Cars. Kindle Direct Publishing 2022. e-book and paperback.
50. Paintings by Kerry Atkinson. 2022. Kindle Direct Publishing 2022. e-book and paperback.
51. Samuel Beckett and Bob Dylan – living in a Shakespearean era. Kindle Direct Publishing 2022. e-book and paperback.
52. Paintings and sculptures by Kerry Atkinson 2023. Kindle Direct Publishing 2023. e-book and paperback.
53. Ten influential European paintings. Kindle Direct Publishing 2023. e-book and paperback
54. The Pillars of Rock 'N Roll. Kindle Direct Publishing 2024. e-book and paperback
55. Early 20th Century Western paintings - a smorgasbord of color and radical shapes. Kindle Direct Publishing 2024. e-book
56. Insects and other wildlife included in Dutch flower paintings from the Dutch golden age. Kindle Direct Publishing 2024. e-book and paperback

Quotation from a song by The Grateful Dead

"One pill makes you larger

And one pill makes you small

And the ones that mother gives you

Don't do anything at all"

From the song White Rabbit sung by Grace Slick with The Grateful Dead on their album Surrealistic Pillow released by RCA Records in 1967

Table of Contents

1. Author's preface

Check point inhibitors are a new class of drug. Cancers suppress the immune system, removing a mechanism to control them. Check point inhibitors, however, inhibit this suppression, freeing the immune system to react against the cancer.

Check point inhibitors approved by the USAFood and Drug Administration (FDA) thus far are all monoclonal antibodies and their use is a form of immunotherapy.

The FDA has approved three different categories of check point inhibitors (CIs). These are PD-1 inhibitors (Nivolumab, Pembrolizumab, Cemiplimab and Dostarlimab), PDL-1 inhibitors (Atezolimumab, Durvalumab, Avelumab), and CTLA-4 inhibitors (Ipilimumab and Tremelimumab). This book describes the features of check point inhibitors that have been approved for therapeutic use by the USA Food and Drug Administration.

These drugs have markedly changed the treatment outcomes of a number of diseases, most notably melanoma.

Since they release the T cells in the body from tumor-induced suppression, it is not surprising that the T cells can then also attack normal tissues, causing immune-mediated pneumonitis, immune-mediated nephritis, immune-mediated colitis, immune-mediated endocrinopathies and immune-mediated dermatitis. These complications can be severe, and in some cases fatal.

Each check point inhibitor has been FDA-approved for more than one disease. One indicator of how successful check point inhibitors have become is the fact that one of them - pembrolizumab (KEYTRUDA) - manufactured by Merck, has received FDA approval for its use in 17 different malignant diseases. Many of the FDA approvals have been in conjunction with the current cytotoxic drug/s used for each specific malignancy.

The comprehensive understanding of the biology of normal human cells and that of malignant human cells over the last seven decades has led to the development of a large number of new therapeutic agents. Foremost among the beneficiaries of this is medical oncology. When I trained in medical oncology at the Royal Marsden Hospital in 1972 – 1976 all the drugs available were organic chemicals and were known as cytotoxic chemotherapeutic agents. In four diseases they were very effective – even curative. These diseases were childhood (but not adult) acute lymphoblastic leukemia, advanced Hodgkin lymphoma, testicular carcinoma (even if metastatic to the brain) and choriocarcinoma. However, for most other cancers they had little efficacy and many side-effects. The situation today is quite different because of the elucidation over the last seven decades of the biology of normal human cells and that of malignant human cells. This understanding has provided a large number of drug targets, which researchers have been quick to exploit and develop new drugs based on these targets.

One group of drugs, designed as a result of the new understanding of malignant cells are check point inhibitors. Eight of these have been approved by the FDA for the treatment of a number of different cancers, and while not yet curative, they have significantly resulted in improved outcome of these cancers. They are the focus of this book.

Please note:

The text of the FDA HIGHLIGHTS OF PRESCRIBING INFORMATION for the drugs described in detail in this book is taken verbatim from the FDA document specific for the drug described. Additionally, I have included the Mechanism of Action of each drug and the Clinical Trial information of each drug. These latter data are taken verbatim from the FDA FULL PRESCRIBING INFORMATION of each drug. Both the FDA Highlights of Prescribing and the FDA Full Prescribing Information are in the public domain

I have added clinical information throughout the book to give information about some adverse clinical events caused by the drugs described. I have made it clear in each instance that this information is NOT in the FDA documents by putting all such additions in parentheses and have put the text in italics.

I have also put in bold font some headings in the FDA documents that I think are particularly important for the clinician using these drugs to be aware of.

There are three numbering systems in this book: firstly, that of the Table of Contents, which lists chronologically each major section of the book; secondly, that used in the FDA Highlights of Prescribing document; and thirdly, that used in the FDA Full Prescribing Information document. I have not altered the numbering in the case of the two latter documents. Some sections or subsections were omitted from the full FDA Prescribing Information. Thus, the numbering system within the FDA documents for each of the four drugs described is not always chronological.

2. Introduction to cancer treatment and immune check pointdrugs

The five major biomedical revolutions of the second half of the 20th century are

The production of monoclonal antibodies

The discovery of DNA and how it, RNA and amino acids make proteins

Epigenetics and the posttranslational modification of proteins

The discovery of cell signalling pathways

The cloning of the human genome

Cancer treatment overall includes medical oncology, radiation oncology and surgical oncology. Medical oncology has been the main beneficiary of the new medications developed as a result of the detailed knowledge of cell biology that has occurred over the last seven decades.

These discoveries in cellular and molecular biology have revealed to scientists appropriate targets for new drugs and the number that have been produced in the last 30 years, and that are still being produced, has hugely enlarged the therapeutic pharmacopeia, producing treatments - even cures - for diseases that were previously untreatable. The majority of these new treatments have been derived because of much more detailed knowledge about how human cells work. They are therefore known as biological treatments, often abbreviated to biologics. An example of a biologic is the monoclonal antibody rituximab which reacts specifically with the CD20 antigen present only on B cells, but with no other targets.

In addition, other agents that react specifically with one, or at most, several, targets are chemically synthesized: an example is imatinib, which is specific for the tyrosine kinase (TK) domain in abl (the Abelson proto-oncogene), c-kit and PDGF-R (platelet-derived growth factor receptor). Another example is sonedegib, which inhibits activation of the intracellular Hedgehog signalling pathway.

The inclusion of therapeutic agents is based on their specificity for a given target. For example, interleukin 2 (IL-2) would not be included since it has a range of biological activities including the proliferation of T cells, the generation of T cell cytotoxic responses and the recall of cytotoxic T cell memory. Likewise, interferon-alpha (IFN-α) would not be included since its functions include antiviral activity, antiproliferative activity, NK cell activation, cytokine induction, and interferon-stimulated gene-induction activity. This exclusion applies even though each are made constitutively in the body in response to specific diseases: they are biologic agents, but their targets are broad.

This series of books explains what the new treatments are, how they work and how they compare, and interact with, conventional treatment. It is important to state that no book in this series makes specific treatment recommendations for any of the diseases covered: such decisions should be initiated and reviewed by an appropriate medical specialist. Much information on each disease is available free of charge from Wikipedia (wikipedia.org), from postgraduate textbooks on each disease and from UpToDate.com: the latter website gives information for patients and caregivers free of charge but a subscription is required for more detailed information. Rather, the purpose of this series of books is to give information on newly developed biological and specifically designed treatments and their mechanism of action, hopefully enabling the reader to get a handle on these extensive additions to the medical pharmacopeia.

A distinction is made between monoclonal antibodies (the mabs) as “immunotherapy”, the small specifically designed inhibitory molecules (the nibs, which are protein kinase inhibitors) and the receptor blocking agents (the cepts) – the latter sometimes known as decoy receptors. However, since each category of drug has been developed from the comprehensive knowledge of human cell biology discovered over the past seven decades, and as each drug in each category is exquisitely targeted to a specific epitope on a cell surface protein (the mabs), the inhibition of a specific intracellular enzyme process (the nibs), or the blocking of a specific cell surface receptor (the cepts) I prefer to combine the mabs, the nibs and the cepts in the single category of targeted biological treatments. An example from each category are rituximab, imatinib and etanercept.

A fourth type of biological targeted agents has now been FDA-approved for therapeutic use – sonidegib and vismodegib – both of which specifically target the intracellular Hedgehog pathway and are now both FDA-approved for treatment of basal cell carcinoma of the skin.

A fifth type of biological targeted agents approved by the FDA for treatment in a large number of different cancers are the check point inhibitors, which decrease the suppression of T cell activity common in all cancers, thus enabling the patients' own T cells to act against their cancer. Mice with the CTLA-4 gene removed (e.g. CTLA-4 knockout mice) develop severe autoimmune disease, with diffuse infiltration of T cells in multiple organs and fatal enterocolitis. In clinical medicine these agents have made significant improvements in the outcome of a number of malignancies, notably in malignant melanoma. Check point inhibitor therapy is known as a form of cancer immunotherapy, since all check point inhibitors developed thus far are monoclonal antibodies. This therapy targets immune checkpoints, which are key regulators of the immune system, that when stimulated, can dampen the immune response to an immunologic stimulus such as a tumor antigen. The first anti-cancer drug targeting an immune check point was ipilimumab, a CTLA4 blocker approved in the United States in 2011.

Currently approved check point inhibitors target the molecules CTLA4, PD-1, and PD-L1. PD-1 is the transmembrane programmed cell death 1 protein (also called PDCD1 and CD279), which interacts with PD-L1 (PD-1 ligand 1, or CD274). PD-L1 on the cell surface binds to PD-1 on an immune cell surface, which inhibits immune cell activity. Among PD-L1 functions is a key regulatory role on T cell activities. It appears that cancers upregulate the expression of PD-L1 on the cell surface, which in turn may inhibit T cells that might otherwise attack the cancer. Check point inhibitors bind to either PD-1 or PD-L1 and therefore block this interaction, thus enabling the patient's T cells to attack the tumor cells.

PD-1 is a cell surface receptor on T cells and B cells that has a role in regulating the immune system's response to the cells of the human body by down-regulating the immune system and promoting self-tolerance by suppressing T cell inflammatory activity. This prevents autoimmune diseases, but it can also prevent the immune system from killing cancer cells.

Figure 1. Structure of PD-1 (programmed death protein 1, aka PDC-1: programmed cell death protein-1.

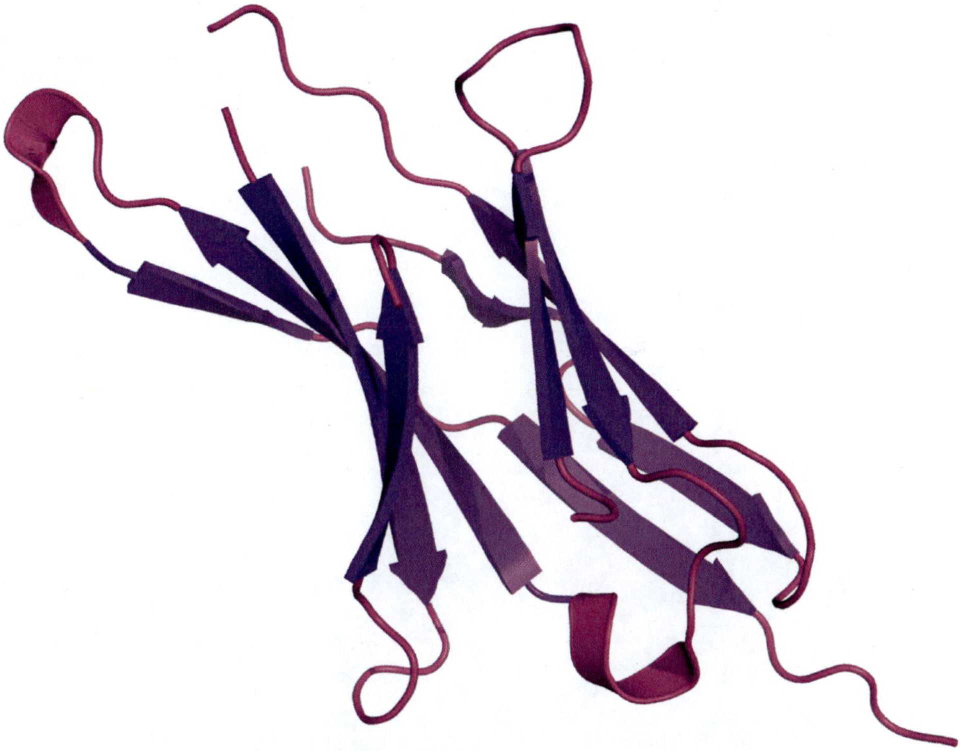

This image is by Fvasconcellos (talk · contribs) - From PDB entry 3RRQ., Public Domain, https://commons.wikimedia.org/w/index.php?curid=61346859; https://en.wikipedia.org/wiki/Programmed_cell_death_protein_1#/media/File:PD-1_ribbon_3RRQ.png. The copyright holder of this work has released this work into the public domain.

Figure 2. Crystal structure of CTLA4 as published in the Protein Data Bank (PDB: 1DQT

Cytotoxic T-lymphocyte associated protein 4, (CTLA-4) also known as CD152 (cluster of differentiation 152), is a protein receptor that functions as an immune checkpoint and downregulates immune responses. CTLA-4 is constitutively expressed in regulatory T cells but only upregulated in conventional T cells after activation – a phenomenon which is particularly notable in cancers.[5] It acts as an "off" switch when bound to CD80 or CD86 on the surface of antigen-presenting cell)s.

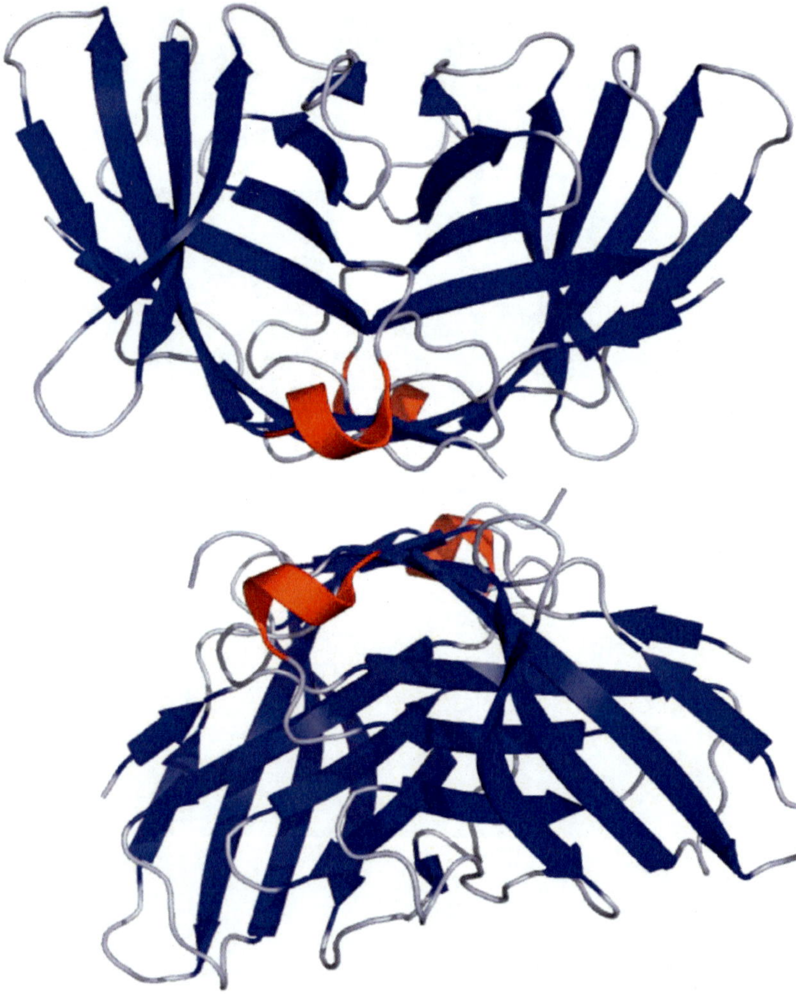

This image is by Ramin Herati - Created from PDB 1DQT and rendered by me using Pymol, Public Domain, https://commons.wikimedia.org/w/index.php?curid=1450193; https://en.wikipedia.org/wiki/Cytotoxic_T-lymphocyte_associated_protein_4#/media/File:CTLA4_Crystal_Structure.rsh.png. the copyright holder of this work, release this work into the public domain. No changes were made to this image.

Figure 3. Binding interactions between the B7 family of ligands on antigen-binding cells (APCs) and their receptors on activated T cells.

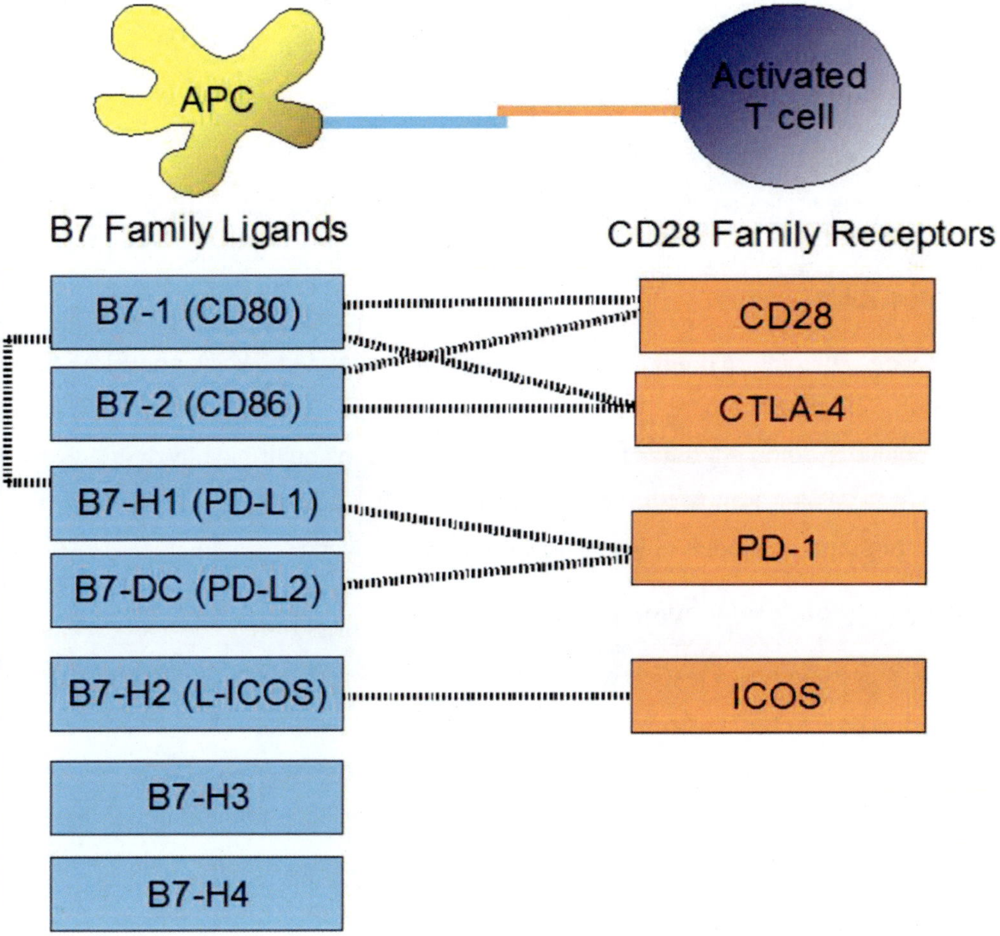

This image is by The Immunologist - Own work, CC0, https://commons.wikimedia.org/w/index.php?curid=7741911; https://en.wikipedia.org/wiki/PD-L1#/media/File:B7_family_ligands_and_CD28_family_receptors.JPG. This file is made available under the Creative Commons CC0 1.0 Universal Public Domain Dedication. No changes were made to this image.

There is now a sixth type of biological targeted therapeutic agents that have been approved by the FDA for therapeutic use: chimeric antigen receptor modified (CAR) T cells. The first such agent – tisagenlecleucel – was approved by the USA FDA in 2017 for use in people with acute lymphoblastic leukemia. CAR T cells are an innovative cellular immunotherapeutic approach that involves genetic modification of autologous T cells such that they express target tumor antigen/s as well as a component of the T cell activation pathway – the CD3 zeta chain. T cell surface glycoprotein CD3 zeta chain, also known as T cell receptor T3 zeta chain or CD247, together with T cell receptor alpha/beta and gamma/delta heterodimers and CD3-gamma, -delta, and -epsilon, forms the T cell receptor-CD3 complex. The zeta chain plays an important role in coupling antigen recognition to several intracellular signal-transduction pathways. Upon recognition of the tumor antigen, the transduced T cells become cytotoxic and destroy the tumor cell.

CAR T cells represent the second type of cellular therapy to be therapeutically successful. The first successful cellular therapy was the use of hematopoietic stem cells, introduced in the late 1960s, which offered curative treatment for diseases that were not curable by any other type of therapy.

This new drug discovery phenomenon is a therapeutic tsunami which shows no sign of slowing. The pharmacopeia has increased enormously and all medical students should consider doing a Master's degree or a PhD in molecular biology. It is only by working in a cellular or molecular biology laboratory (usually combined) that one can really understand how each of these new medications work.

3.The biology of normal human cells

To fully understand how these new therapeutic agents work it is useful to understand how cells work – in particular, what signalling pathways they use. Normal cells and cells in tissues affected by non- diseases use signalling pathways often different from those used by cells. All human cells are derived from a single totipotent stem cell which is produced by the fusion of a single sperm with a single ovum. This totipotent stem cell has all the genes on its chromosomes responsible for the future growth and development of the fetus, including reproductive capacity. Cell biology is concerned with the physiological properties, metabolic processes, signalling pathways, life cycle, chemical composition and interactions of cells with their environment. Cell biology involves genetics, biochemistry, molecular
biology, immunology and cytochemistry. Human cells are eukaryotes - they contain organelles. The generalized structure of a eukaryotic cell is shown in Figure 4.

Figure 4. A diagram of a mammalian cell

This image has been released into the public domain by its author, LadyofHats (Mariana Ruiz). Source: own work using Adobe Illustrator. Image renamed from Image:Animal cell structure.svg.
https://commons.wikimedia.org/wiki/File:Animal_cell_structure_en.svg. No changes have been made to this image.

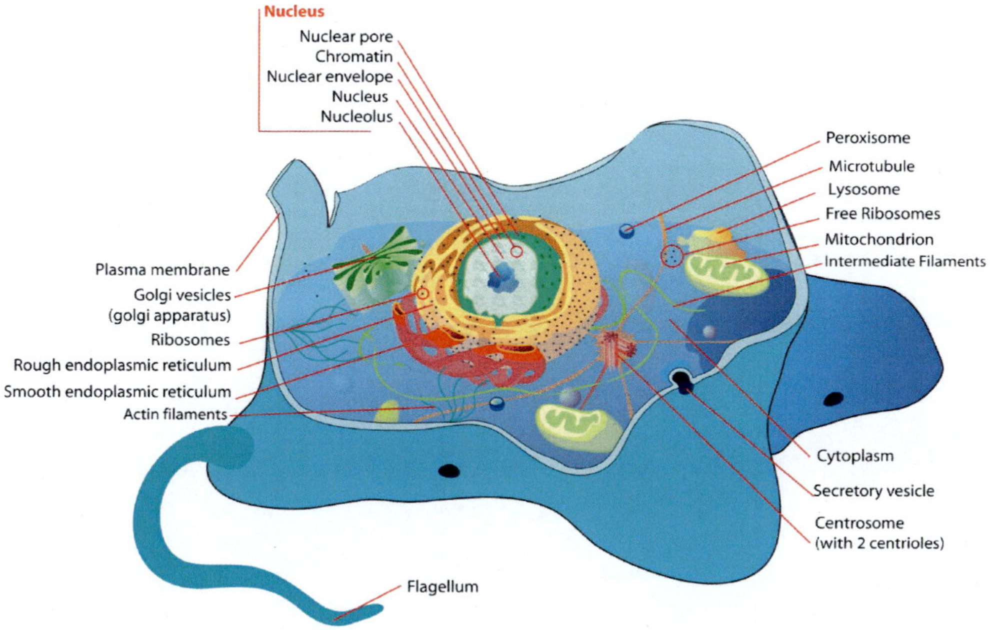

Most of the processes of eukaryotic cells are performed by a mixture of small organic molecules, inorganic ions, hormones and water. Approximately 75-85% of the cell's volume is due to water making it an indispensable solvent as a result of its polarity and structure. The shape of cells are generally round and spherical or oval.

The main constituents of the cell include proteins and lipids which are either free-flowing or membrane-bound, along with different internal compartments known as organelles. The cytoplasm is all of the material within a cell, enclosed by the cell membrane, except for the cell nucleus. The material inside the nucleus and contained within the nuclear membrane is termed the nucleoplasm. A cell's DNA, contained on the cell's chromosomes, is located within the cell's nucleus. The main components of the cytoplasm are cytosol – a gel-like substance, the organelles – the cell's internal sub-structures - and various cytoplasmic inclusions. Cell are composed of hydrophilic and hydrophobic regions. The hydrophilic regions of the cell are on both the inside and outside of the cell, while the hydrophobic regions are within the phospholipid bilayer of the cell membrane. A diagram of a mammalian cell membrane is shown in Figure 5. This shows the detailed diagram of lipid bilayer cell membrane. The cell membrane, also called the plasma membrane or plasmalemma, biological molecules, primarily proteins and lipids, which are involved in a vast array of cellular processes. It also serves as the attachment point for both the intracellular cytoskeleton and, if present, the cell wall.

Figure 5.

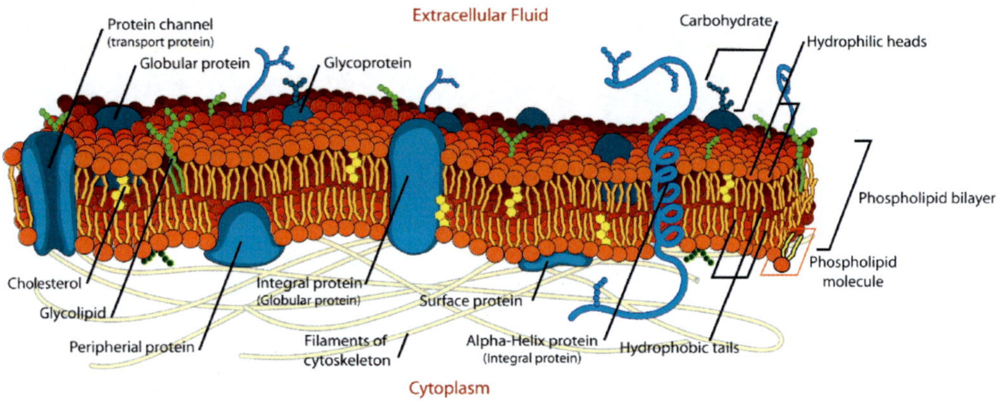

This image has been released into the public domain by its author, LadyofHats (Mariana Ruiz). Source: Own work. Image renamed from File:Cell membrane detailed diagram.svg. https://commons.wikimedia.org/wiki/File:Cell_membrane_detailed_diagram_en.svg. No changes have been made to this image.

In order for molecules to participate in reactions within the cell, they need to be able to cross this membrane layer to get into the cell. They accomplish this process of gaining access to the cell via osmotic pressure, diffusion, concentration gradients, and membrane channels. Inside the cell are extensive internal suB cellular membrane-bounded compartments called organelles.

Figure 6. Some of the cell surface proteins and internal signalling pathways of a normal human cell.

This image is in the public domain in the United States because it is a work prepared by an officer or employee of the United States Government as part of that person's official duties under the terms of Title 17, Chapter 1, Section 105 of the US Code. Source: http://dir.niehs.nih.gov/dirlst/imagemap/cell.jpg. https://commons.wikimedia.org/wiki/File:NIEHScell.jpg. No changes have been made to this image.

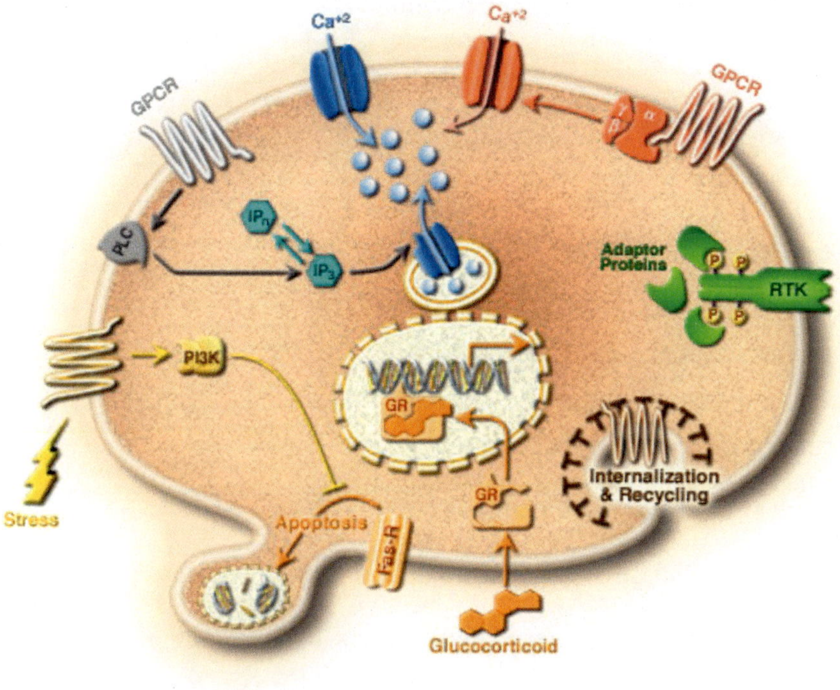

Cell growth pertains to the increase in the number of cells present in an organism as it grows and develops; in order for the organism to grow the number of cells present must increase. To enable cell growth and development the cell goes through the steps of the cell cycle: DNA replication, cell division, regeneration, specialization, and cell death. The cell cycle is divided into four distinct phases, G1, S, G2, and M. The G phases (cell growth) make up approximately 95% of the cycle. After proliferation cells then differentiate to become specialized in order to form specialized tissues, then organs and ultimately systems. The G phases along with the S phase – DNA replication, damage and repair - are considered to be the interphase portion of the cycle. While the M phase (mitosis and cytokinesis) is the cell division portion of the cycle. The cell cycle is regulated by a series of signalling factors and complexes such as cyclin-dependent kinases and p53. When the cell has completed its growth process, and if it is found to be damaged or altered, it undergoes cell death, either by apoptosis or necrosis, in order to eliminate the threat it can cause to the organism's survival.

Essential cell processes include

Active transport and passive transport – the movement of molecules into and out of cells

Adhesion - holding cells and tissues together

Cell movement - chemotaxis, contraction and cilia

Cell signalling - regulation of cell behaviour by signals from outside and inside the cell

Division – the process by which cells reproduce either by mitosis (to produce clones of the parent cell) or meiosis (to produce haploid gametes either male [sperm)] or female [ova]) dependent on the gender of the organism

DNA repair - cell death and cell senescence

Metabolism - glycolysis, respiration, photosynthesis, and chemosynthesis

Signal transduction - the process by which the activities in the cell are regulated

Transcription and mRNA splicing - gene expression

Three of the most important processes – signal transduction, gene expression and apoptosis (also known as programmed cell death) - are described furtherl below. Some of the most important pathways for understanding the basis of targeted therapies, such as the pathways for angiogenesis, interleukin (IL) 4, IL-12 and IL-23 and the TNF pathways are described in chapters dealing with the therapeutic use of molecules involved in these pathways.

Signal transduction and cell signalling pathways

Signal transduction is the process by which a chemical or physical signal is transmitted through a cell as a series of molecular events, most commonly protein phosphorylation catalysed by protein kinases, which ultimately results in a cellular response. Proteins responsible for detecting stimuli such as ligands are termed receptors The changes elicited by ligand binding to a receptor give rise to a biochemical cascade otherwise known as a signalling path.

When signalling pathways interact with one another they form networks, which allow cellular responses to be coordinated, often by combinatorial signalling events. At the molecular level, such responses include changes in the transcription or translation of genes, and post-translational and conformational changes in proteins, as well as changes in their location. These molecular events are the basic mechanisms controlling cell growth, proliferation, metabolism and many other processes. In multicellular organisms, signal transduction pathways have evolved to regulate cell communication in a wide variety of ways.

Each component (or node) of a signalling pathway is classified according to the role it plays with respect to the initial stimulus. Ligands are termed first messengers, while receptors are the signal transducers, which then activate primary effectors. Such effectors are often linked to second messengers, which can activate secondary effectors, and so on. Depending on the efficiency of the nodes, a signal can be amplified (a concept known as signal gain), so that one signalling molecule can generate a response involving hundreds to millions of molecules With the advent of computational biology, the analysis of signalling pathways and networks has become an essential tool to understand cellular functions and disease, including signalling rewiring mechanisms underlying responses to acquired drug resistance.

Ligands

The majority of signal transduction pathways involve the binding of signalling molecules, known as ligands, to receptors that trigger events inside the cell. The binding of a signalling molecule with a receptor causes a change in the conformation of the receptor, known as receptor activation. Most ligands are soluble molecules from the extracellular medium which bind to cell surface receptors. These include growth factors, cytokines and neurotransmitters. Components of the extracellular matrix such as fibronectin and hyaluronan can also bind to such receptors (integrins and CD44, respectively). In addition, some molecules such as steroid hormones are lipid-soluble and thus cross the plasma membrane to reach nuclear receptors.

Some receptors such as HER2/neu are capable of ligand-independent activation when overexpressed or mutated. This leads to constitutive activation of the pathway, which may or may not be overturned by compensation mechanisms. In the case of HER2, which acts as a dimerization partner of other EGFRs, constitutive activation leads to hyperproliferation and cancer – primarily some cases of breast cancer and gastric cancer (HER2/neu is also known as receptor tyrosine-protein kinase erbB-2, CD340, proto-oncogene Neu and ERBB2). A ribbon diagram of the Fab fragment of trastuzumab, a monoclonal antibody, bound to the extracellular domain of HER2 is shown in Figure 7.

Figure 7. A ribbon diagram of the Fab fragment of trastuzumab

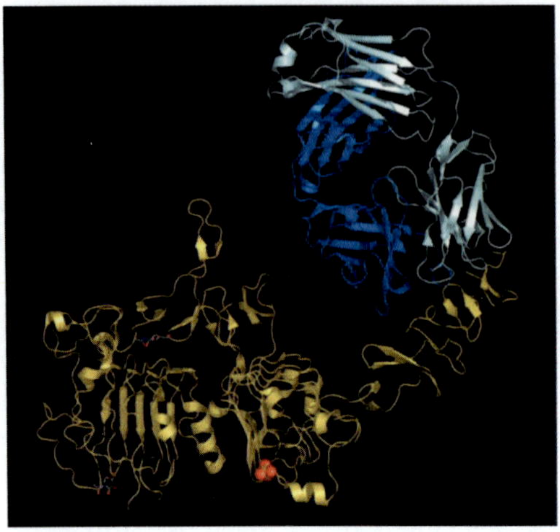

Ribbon diagram of the Fab fragment of trastuzumab, a monoclonal antibody, bound to the extracellular domain of HER2. Legend: Trastuzumab Fab fragment, heavy chain ; Trastuzumab Fab fragment, light chain ; HER2, extracellular domain

Extracellular receptors, ligand binding, messengers and adaptor proteins

Extracellular receptors are integral transmembrane proteins that span the plasma membrane of the cell, with one part of the receptor on the outside of the cell and the other on the inside. Signal transduction occurs as a result of a ligand binding to the outside region of the receptor (the ligand does not pass through the membrane). Ligand-receptor binding induces a change in the conformation of the inside part of the receptor, a process sometimes called "receptor activation". This results in either the activation of an enzyme domain of the receptor or the exposure of a binding site for other intracellular signalling proteins within the cell, eventually propagating the signal through the cytoplasm.

In mammalian cells most intracellular proteins activated by a ligand/receptor interaction possess an enzymatic activity; examples include tyrosine kinases and phosphatases. Often such enzymes are covalently linked to the receptor. Some of them create second messengers such as cyclic AMP and IP3, the latter controlling the release of intracellular calcium stores into the cytoplasm. Other activated proteins interact with adaptor proteins that facilitate signalling protein interactions and coordination of signalling complexes necessary to respond to a particular stimulus. Enzymes and adaptor proteins are both responsive to various second messenger molecules.

Many adaptor proteins and enzymes activated as part of signal transduction possess specialized protein domains that bind to specific secondary messenger molecules. For example, calcium ions bind to the EF hand domains of calmodulin, allowing it to bind and activate calmodulin-dependent kinase.

The following major extracellular receptor/ligand binding pathways will be discussed in more detail below:

G protein-coupled receptors

Tyrosine, seronine/threonine- and histidine-specific protein kinases

Integrins

Toll-like receptors

Ligand-gated ion binding channels

G proteins, also known as guanine nucleotide-binding proteins, are a family of proteins that act as molecular switches inside cells, and are involved in transmitting signals from a variety of stimuli outside a cell to its interior. Their activity is regulated by factors that control their ability to bind to and hydrolyze guanosine triphosphate (GTP) to guanosine diphosphate (GDP). When they are bound to GTP, they are 'on', and, when they are bound to GDP, they are 'off'.

They possess seven transmembrane domains and are linked to a heterotrimeric G protein (Figure 8). Beta and gamma subunits of G-protein are shown by blue and red, respectively, in the phosducin transducin beta-gamma complex. (Phosducin binds tightly to the beta gamma subunits (Gt beta gamma) of the heterotrimeric G protein transducin, preventing Gt beta gamma reassociation with Gt alpha-GDP and thereby inhibiting the G-protein cycle).

Figure 8. Ribbon diagram of a G protein

This image has been released into the public domain by its creator, Andrei Lomize, has placed it there. By Andrei Lomize - Own work, Public Domain,

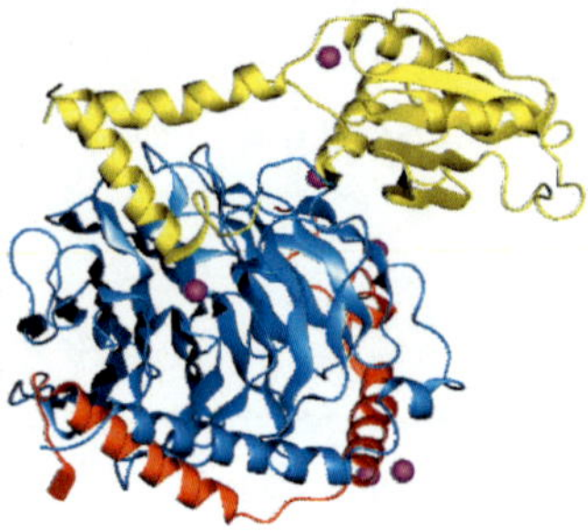

Tyrosine and seronine/threonine-specific protein kinases

Receptor tyrosine kinases (RTKs) are transmembrane proteins with an intracellular kinase domain and an extracellular domain that binds ligands; examples include growth factor receptors such as the insulin receptor. To perform signal transduction, RTKs need to form dimers in the plasma membrane. The dimer is stabilized by ligands binding to the receptor. The interaction between the cytoplasmic domains stimulates the autophosphorylation of tyrosine residues within the intracellular kinase domains of the RTKs, causing conformational changes. Subsequent to this, the receptors' kinase domains are activated, initiating phosphorylation signaling cascades of downstream cytoplasmic molecules that facilitate various cellular processes such as cell differentiation and metabolism. Many serine/threonine and dual-specificity protein kinases are important for signal transduction, either acting downstream of receptor tyrosine kinases, or as membrane-embedded or cell-soluble versions in their own right. The process of signal transduction involves around 560 known protein kinases and pseudokinanases, encoded by the human kinome. The kinome of an organism is the complete set of protein kinases encoded in its genome.

As is the case with GPCRs, proteins that bind GTP play a major role in signal transduction from the activated RTK into the cell. In this case, the G proteins are members of the Ras, Rho, and Raf families, referred to collectively as small G proteins. They act as molecular switches usually tethered to membranes by isoprenyl groups linked to their carboxyl ends. Upon activation, they assign proteins to specific membrane subdomains where they participate in signalling. Activated RTKs in turn activate small G proteins that activate guanine nucleotide exchange factors such as SOS1. Once activated, these exchange factors can activate more small G proteins, thus amplifying the receptor's initial signal. The mutation of certain RTK genes, as with that of GPCRs, can result in the expression of receptors that exist in a constitutively activated state. Such mutated genes may act as oncogenes. An example is the BCR-ABL gene, which is translated to the BCR-ABL protein, a growth factor responsible for the development of chronic myeloid leukemia (CML). The first tyrosine kinase inhibitor developed that was therapeutically successful is imatinib, now routinely used as first-line treatment of CML, obviating the need in many cases of the only curative treatment for CML – allogeneic hematopoietic stem cell transplantaion, a procedure that had a treatment-related mortality of 20-30%.

Integrins

Integrins are produced by a wide variety of cells. They play a role in cell attachment to other cells and the extracellular matrix and in the transduction of signals from extracellular matrix components such as fibronectin and collagen (Figure 9).

Figure 9. An overview of integrin-mediated signal transduction, adapted from Hehlgens et al. (2007).

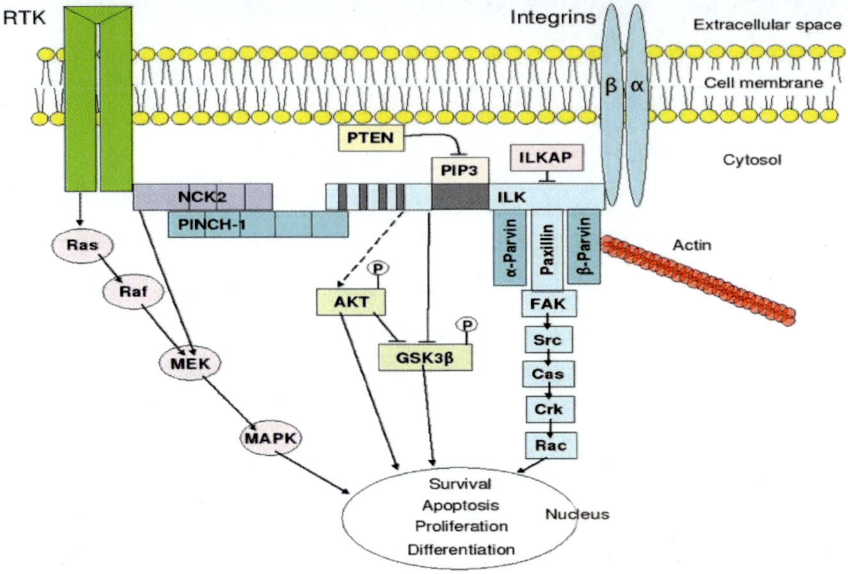

Ligand binding to the extracellular domain of integrins changes the protein's conformation, clustering it at the cell membrane to initiate signal transduction. Integrins lack kinase activity; hence, integrin-mediated signal transduction is achieved through a variety of intracellular protein kinases and adaptor molecules, the main coordinator being integrin-linked kinase. As shown in Figure 7, cooperative integrin-RTK signaling determines the timing of cellular survival, apoptosis, proliferation and differentiation.

Toll-like receptors

When activated, toll-like receptors (TLRs) take adapter molecules within the cytoplasm of cells in order to propagate a signal.

Four adaptor molecules are known to be involved in signalling. These are Myd88, TIRAP, TRIF, and TRAM. These adapter molecules activate other intracellular molecules such as IRAK1, IRAK4, TBK1, and IKKi that amplify the signal, eventually leading to the induction or suppression of genes that cause certain responses. Thousands of genes are activated by TLR signalling, implying that this method constitutes an important gateway for gene modulation.

Messenger systems

First messengers are the signalling molecules (hormones, neurotransmitters and paracrine/autocrine agents) that reach the cell from the extracellular fluid and bind to their specific receptors.

Second messengers are the substances that enter the cytoplasm and act within the cell to trigger a response. Second messengers serve as chemical relays from the plasma membrane to the cytoplasm, thus carrying out intracellular signal transduction.

Calcium

The release of calcium ions from the endoplasmic reticulum into the cytosol results in its binding to signalling proteins that are then activated. It is then sequestered in the smooth endoplasmic reticulum and the mitochondria. Calcium is used in many processes including muscle contraction, neurotransmitter release from nerve endings, and cell migration. The three main pathways that lead to its activation are GPCR pathways, RTK pathways, and gated ion channels. It regulates proteins either directly or by binding to an enzyme.

Cellular responses

Gene activations and metabolism alterations are examples of cellular responses to extracellular stimulation that require signal transduction. Gene activation leads to further cellular effects, since the products of responding genes include instigators of activation. Transcription factors produced as a result of a signal transduction cascade can activate even more genes. Hence, an initial stimulus can trigger the expression of a large number of genes, leading to physiological events. Examples are the increased uptake of glucose from the blood stream and the migration of neutrophils to sites of infection.

Mammalian cells require stimulation for cell division and survival. In the absence of growth factor, apoptosis (programmed cell death – see below) ensues. Such requirements for extracellular stimulation are necessary for controlling cell behavior. Signal transduction pathways are perceived to be so central to biological processes that a large number of diseases are attributed to their dysregulation. Three basic types of signals determine cellular growth:

Stimulatory signals (growth factors)

Transcription-dependent response

Steroids are an example of this. They bind DNA, which needs to be transcribed. The produced mRNA needs to be translated, and the produced protein/peptide can undergo posttranslational modification (PMT).

Transcription-independent response

Epidermal growth factor (EGF) is an example. It binds to the epidermal growth factor receptor (EGFR), which causes dimerization and autophosphorylation of the EGFR, which in turn activates the intracellular signalling pathway.

Inhibitory signals (cell-cell contact)

Permissive signals (cell-matrix interactions)

The combination of these signals are integrated in an altered cytoplasmic machinery which leads to altered cell behaviour.

Major cell signalling pathways

The following are some of the major cell signalling pathways, demonstrating how ligands binding to their receptors can affect second messengers and eventually result in altered cellular responses.

MAPK/ERK pathway: a pathway that couples intracellular responses to the binding of growth factors to cell surface receptors. This pathway is very complex and includes many protein components. In many cell types, activation of this pathway promotes cell division, and many forms of cancer are associated with aberrations in it.

cAMP-dependent pathway: cAMP works by activating protein kinase A (PKA, cAMP-dependent protein kinase. Further effects depend mainly on cAMP-dependent protein kinase, which vary based on the type of cell involved.

IP3/DAG pathway: PLC cleaves the phospholipid phosphatidylinositol 4,5-bisphosphate (PIP2), yielding diacyl glycerol (DAG) and inositol 1,4,5-triphosphate (IP3). DAG remains bound to the membrane, and IP3 is released as a soluble structure into the cytosol. IP3 then diffuses through the cytosol to bind to IP3 receptors, particular calcium channels in the endoplasmic reticulum (ER). These channels are specific to calcium and allow the passage of only calcium to move through. This causes the cytosolic concentration of calcium to increase, in turn precipitating a cascade of intracellular changes and activity. In addition, calcium and DAG together work to activate PKC, which then phosphorylates other molecules, leading to altered cellular activity.

DNA, RNA and genes

DNA is a molecule composed of two chains that coil around each other to form a double helix carrying the genetic instructions used in the growth, development, functioning, and reproduction of all known organisms and many viruses. DNA and ribonucleic acid (RNA) are nucleic acids. Nucleic acids, together with proteins, lipids and complex carbohydrates (polysaccharides), are one of the four major types of macromolecules that are essential for all known forms of life.

The two DNA strands are also known as polynucleotides as they are composed of simpler monomeric units called nucleotides. Each nucleotide is composed of one of four nitrogen-containing nucleobases (cytosine [C], guanine [G], adenine [A] or thymine [T]), a sugar called deoxyribose, and a phosphate group.

Figure 10 is a graphic of DNA replication. The nitrogenous bases of the two separate polynucleotide strands are bound together, according to base pairing rules (A with T and C with G), with hydrogen bonds to make double-stranded DNA in a helical form.

Figure 10. A graphic of DNA replication.

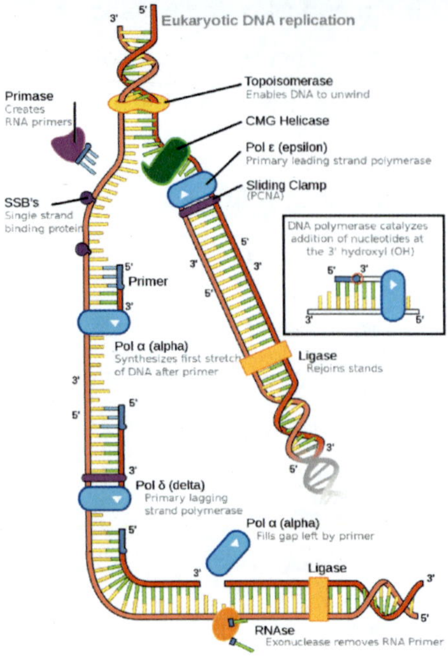

Genes

A gene is a sequence of nucleotides in DNA or RNA that codes for a molecule that has a function. Genes are contained on the chromosomes in the cell nucleus. During gene expression, the DNA is first copied into RNA. The RNA can be directly functional or be the intermediate template for a protein that performs a function. A chromosome consists of a long strand of DNA containing many genes. A human chromosome can have up to 500 million base pairs of DNA with thousands of genes. Gene expression is the process by which information from a gene is used in the synthesis of a functional gene product. These products are often proteins, When the end-product is a protein, genes are first transcribed into RNA, and this transcript is then translated into protein. Several steps in the gene expression process may be modulated, including transcription, RNA splicing, translation and post-translational modification of the protein. Gene regulation gives the cell control over structure and function, and is the basis for cellular differentiation, morphogenesis and the versatility and adaptability of any organism.

Genes are expressed by being transcribed into RNA, and this transcript may then be translated into protein.

Figure 11. Diagram showing how translation of messenger RNA and protein synthesis takes place in ribosomes.

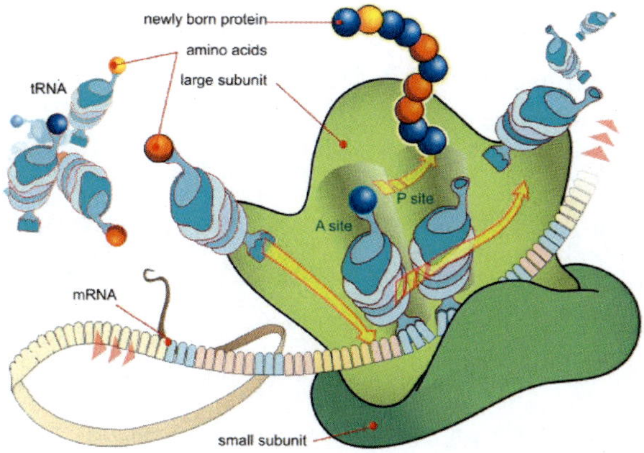

Protein folding

A polypeptide (protein) folds into its characteristic and functional three-dimensional structure from a random coil. Each protein exists as an unfolded polypeptide or random coil when translated from a sequence of messenger (m) RNA into a linear chain of amino acids. Amino acids interact with each other to produce a well-defined three-dimensional structure.

Figure 12 shows a protein before (left) and after (right) folding

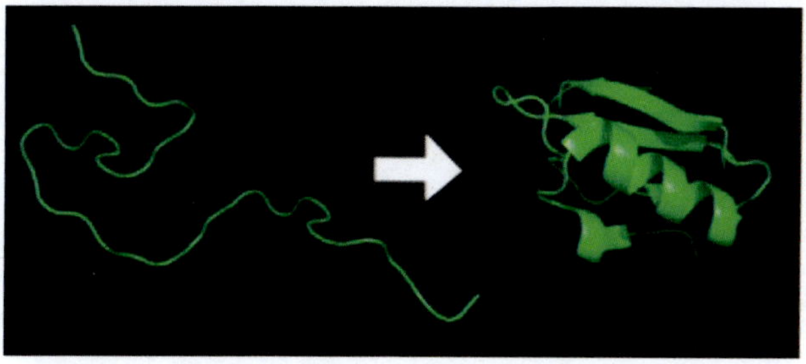

4. The biology of malignant human cells

Defects in genes (DNA), epigenetic factors and mismatch repair systems can all cause human cells to become malignant.

Genes

Malignant human cells have an abnormality of their genetic systems, and differ in this regard to abnormal, but non-malignant, as well as to normal human cells. Carcinogenesis is the formation of a cancer, whereby normal cells are transformed into cancer cells. The process is characterized by changes at the cellular, genetic, and epigenetic levels and abnormal cell division. Cell division is a physiological process that occurs in almost all tissues and under a variety of circumstances. Normally the balance between proliferation and programmed cell death, in the form of apoptosis, is maintained to ensure the integrity of tissues and organs. According to the prevailing accepted theory of carcinogenesis, the somatic mutation theory, mutations in DNA and epimutations that lead to cancer disrupt these orderly processes by disrupting the programming regulating the processes, upsetting the normal balance between proliferation and cell death. This results in uncontrolled cell division and the evolution of those cells by natural selection in the body. Only certain mutations lead to cancer whereas the majority of mutations do not.

A series of several mutations to certain classes of genes is usually required before a normal cell will transform into a malignant cell.

In order for a normal cell to transform into a malignant cell, the genes that regulate cell growth and differentiation must be altered.

The affected genes are divided into two broad categories. Oncogenes are genes that promote cell growth and reproduction. Tumor suppressor genes are genes that inhibit cell division and survival. Malignant transformation can occur through the formation of novel oncogenes, the inappropriate over-expression of normal oncogenes, or by the under-expression or disabling of tumor suppressor genes. Typically, changes in multiple genes are required to transform a normal cell into a cancer cell (Figure 13)

Figure 13 illustrates that cancers are caused by a series of mutations. Each mutation alters the behavior of the cell to some extent.

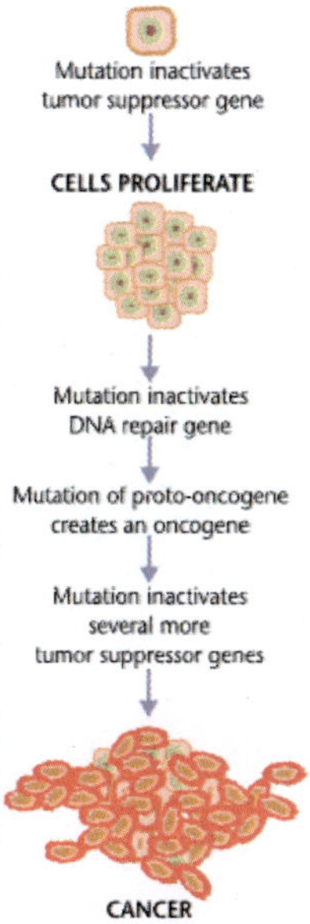

This image is in the public domain because it is a work prepared by an officer or employee of the United States Government as part of that person's official duties under the terms of Title 17, Chapter 1, Section 105 of the US Code. By National Cancer Institute, Public Domain, https://commons.wikimedia.org/w/index.php?curid=1972023. No changes have been made to this image.

The abnormal biological properties of human malignant cells can be summarized as follows:

Acquisition of self-sufficiency in growth signals, leading to unchecked growth.

Loss of sensitivity to anti-growth signals, also leading to unchecked growth.

Loss of capacity for apoptosis, allowing growth despite genetic errors and external anti-growth signals.

Loss of capacity for senescence, leading to limitless replicative potential (immortality).

Acquisition of sustained angiogenesis, allowing the tumor to grow beyond the limitations of passive nutrient diffusion.

Acquisition of ability to invade neighbouring tissues, the defining property of invasive carcinoma.

Acquisition of ability to seed metastases at distant sites, a late-appearing property of some malignant tumors (carcinomas or others).

Involved in these steps is

Loss of capacity to repair genetic errors, leading to an increased mutation rate (genomic instability), thus accelerating all the above changes.

Often, the multiple genetic changes that result in cancer may take many years to accumulate. During this time, the biological behavior of the pre-malignant cells slowly changes from the properties of normal cells to those with cancer-like properties (Figure 14).

Figure 14. Tissue can be organized in a continuous spectrum from normal to malignant.

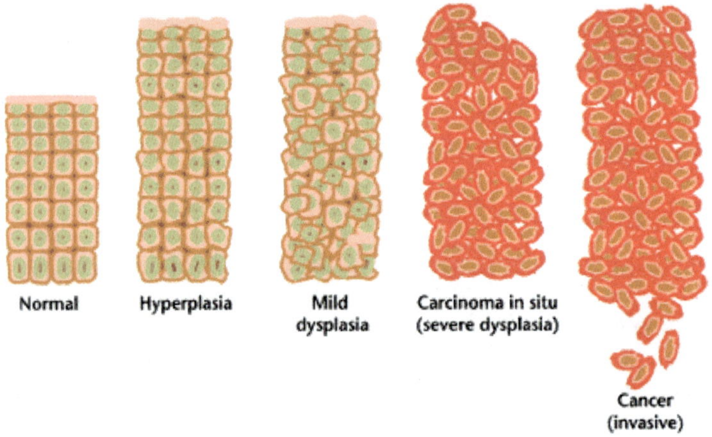

Epigenetic factors also plays a major role in the development of human cancers

Epigenetic modifications to the DNA of cancer cells do not involve a change in the nucleotide sequence, but instead involve a change in the way the genetic code is expressed. Epigenetic alterations may be just as important, or even more important, than genetic mutations in a cell's transformation to malignancy. In malignant cells loss of expression of genes occurs about 10 times more frequently by transcription silencing (caused by epigenetic promoter hypermethylation of CpG islands) than by mutations. In different types of cancer, a variety of epigenetic mechanisms can be perturbed, such as silencing of tumor suppressor genes and activation of oncogenes by altered CpG island methylation patterns, histone modifications, and dysregulation of DNA-binding proteins.

DNA mismatch repair systems

If DNA repair is deficient, DNA damage tends to accumulate. Such excess DNA damage can increase mutational errors during DNA replication. Excess DNA damage can also increase epigenetic alterations due to errors during DNA repair. Such mutations and epigenetic alterations can give rise to malignancy. Germ line mutations in DNA repair genes cause only 2–5% of colon cancer cases. However, altered expression of microRNAs, causing DNA repair deficiencies, are frequently associated with cancers and may be an important causal factor for such cancers.

In non-hereditary cancers, a deficiency in DNA repair is occasionally found to be due to a mutation in a DNA repair gene, but reduced or absent expression of DNA repair genes is much more frequently due to epigenetic alterations that reduce or silence gene expression.

Cancer therapy procedures such as chemotherapy and radiotherapy work by overwhelming the capacity of the malignant cells to repair DNA damage, resulting in their death. Cells that are most rapidly dividing – most typically cancer cells – are preferentially affected. An important side-effect is that other non-cancerous but rapidly dividing cells such as progenitor cells in the gut, skin, and hematopoietic system are also affected. Modern cancer treatments attempt to localize the DNA damage to cells and tissues only associated with cancer, either by physical means (concentrating the therapeutic agent in the region of the tumor) or by biochemical means (exploiting a feature unique to cancer cells in the body).

5. CHECKPOINT INHIBITORS

5.1. PD-1 inhibitors *(1,2)*

5.2. OPDUALAG™ (NIVOLUMAB AND RELATLIMAB-RMBW) injection, for intravenous use. Initial U.S. Approval: 2022

INDICATIONS AND USAGE

OPDUALAG is a combination of nivolumab, a programmed death receptor-1 (PD-1) blocking antibody, and relatlimab, a lymphocyte activation gene-3 (LAG-3) blocking antibody, indicated for the treatment of adult and pediatric patients 12 years of age or older with unresectable or metastatic melanoma.

CLINICAL PHARMACOLOGY

MECHANISM OF ACTION

Relatlimab is a human IgG4 monoclonal antibody that binds to the LAG-3 receptor, blocks interaction with its ligands, including MHC II, and reduces LAG-3 pathway-mediated inhibition of the immune response. Antagonism of this pathway promotes T cell proliferation and cytokine secretion. Binding of the PD-1 ligands, PD-L1 and PD-L2, to the PD-1 receptor found on T cells, inhibits T-cell proliferation and cytokine production. Upregulation of PD-1 ligands occurs in some tumors, and signaling through this pathway can contribute to inhibition of active T-cell immune surveillance of tumors.

Nivolumab is a human IgG4 monoclonal antibody that binds to the PD-1 receptor, blocks interaction with its ligands PD-L1 and PD-L2 and reduces PD-1 pathway-mediated inhibition of the immune response, including the anti-tumor immune response. In syngeneic mouse tumor models, blocking PD-1 activity resulted in decreased tumor growth. The combination of nivolumab (anti-PD-1) and relatlimab (anti-LAG-3) results in increased T-cell activation compared to the activity of either antibody alone. In murine syngeneic tumor models, LAG-3 blockade potentiates the anti-tumor activity of PD-1 blockage, inhibiting tumor growth and promoting tumor regression.

(*Figure 15. Extensive melanoma on a person's chest)*

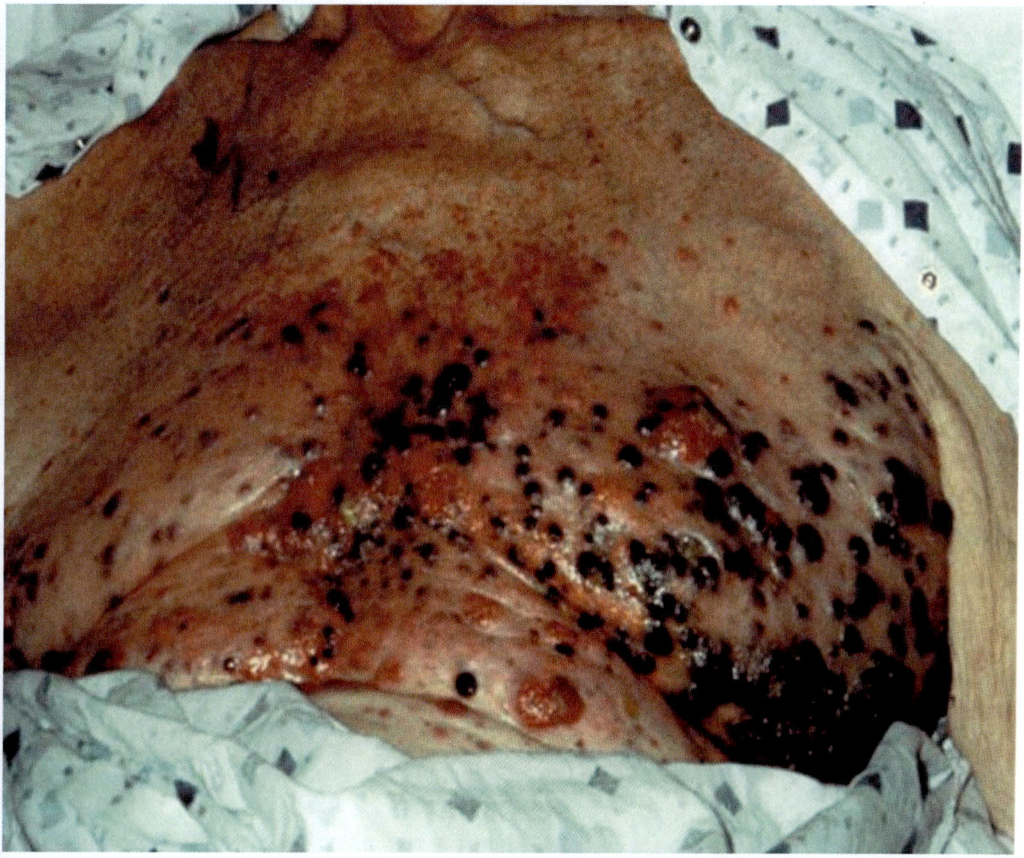

(This image is by CDC/ Carl Washington, M.D., Emory Univ. School of Medicine; Mona Saraiya, MD, MPH - CDC PHIL, #13444, Public Domain, https://commons.wikimedia.org/w/index.php?curid=16362051; en.wikipedia.org/wiki/Melanoma#/media/File:Malignant_melanoma_on_chest.jpg. This image is a work of the Centers for Disease Control and Prevention, part of the United States Department of Health and Human Services, taken or made as part of an employee's official duties. As a work of the U.S. federal government, the image is in the public domain. No changes were made to this image).

DOSAGE AND ADMINISTRATION

• Adult patients and pediatric patients 12 years of age or older who weigh at least 40 kg: 480 mg nivolumab and 160 mg relatlimab intravenously every 4 weeks.

• Administer OPDUALAG as an intravenous infusion over 30 minutes.

•See Full Prescribing Information for dosage modifications for adverse reactions and preparation and administration instructions for the injection

DOSAGE FORMS AND STRENGTHS

• Injection: 240 mg of nivolumab and 80 mg of relatlimab per 20 mL (12 mg and 4 mg per mL) in a single-dose vial.

CONTRAINDICATIONS

• None

WARNINGS AND PRECAUTIONS

• Immune-mediated adverse reactions

o Immune-mediated adverse reactions, which may be severe or fatal, can occur in any organ system or tissue, including the following: immune-mediated pneumonitis, immune-mediated colitis, immune-mediated hepatitis, immune-mediated endocrinopathies, immune-mediated dermatologic adverse reactions, immune-mediated nephritis with renal dysfunction, and immune-mediated myocarditis.

o Monitor for early identification and management.

Evaluate liver enzymes, creatinine, and thyroid function at baseline and periodically during treatment.

o Withhold or permanently discontinue based on severity and type of reaction.

• Infusion-related reactions

Interrupt, slow the rate of infusion, or permanently discontinue OPDUALAG based on severity of reaction.

• Complications of allogeneic hematopoietic atem cell transplantation (HSCT)

Fatal and other serious complications can occur in patient who receive allogeneic HSCT before or after being treated with a PD-1/PD-L1 blocking antibody.

• Embryo-fetal toxicity

Can cause fetal harm. Advise females of reproductive potential of potential risk to a fetus and to use effective contraception.

(Immune-mediated pneumonitis).

(Figure 16. End-stage interstitial lung disease This photo of an autopsy lung with end-stage pulmonary fibrosis).

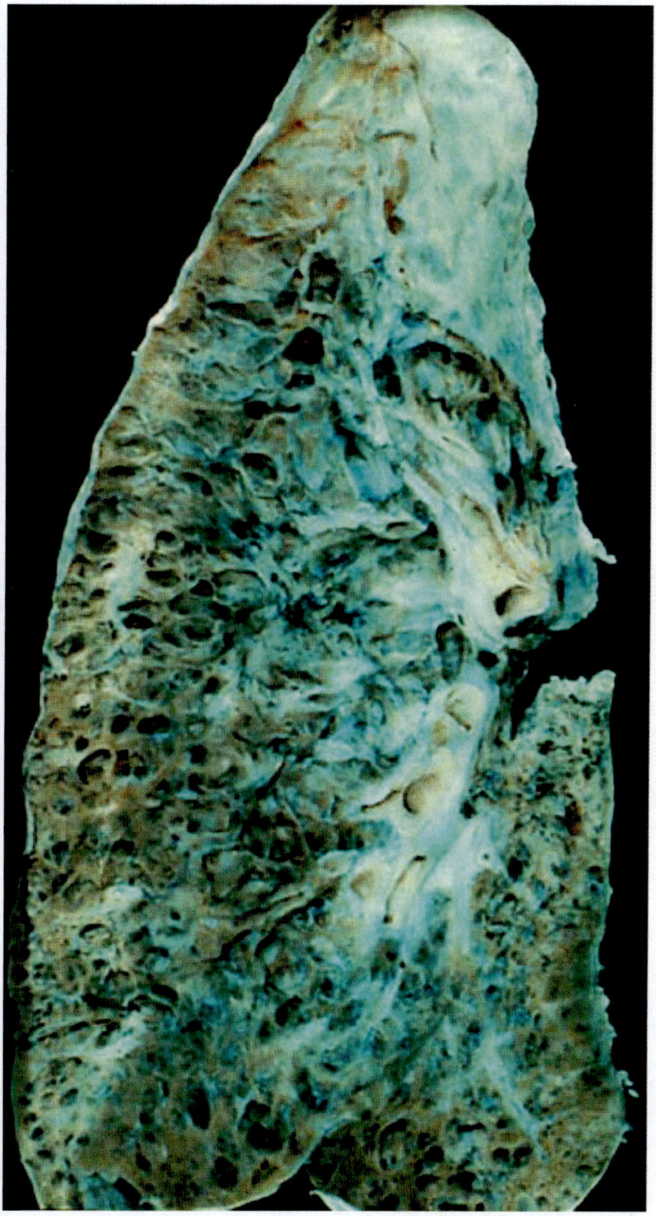

(This image is by http://web2.airmail.net/uthman/specimens/index.html, Public Domain, https://commons.wikimedia.org/w/index.php?curid=841015; en.wikipedia.org/wiki/Interstitial_lung_disease#/media/File:End-stage_interstitial_lung_disease_(honeycomb_lung).jpg. This work has been released into the public domain by its author, Ed Uthman. No changes were made to this mage).

(Immune-mediated colitis)

(Figure 17. Ulceration of the colon in severe colitis)

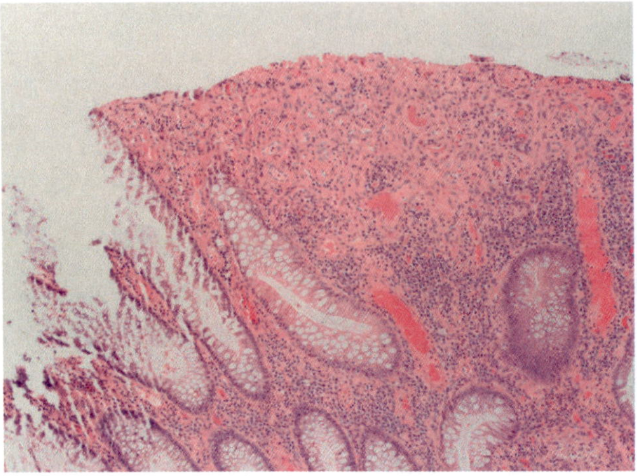

(This image is by Mikael Häggström, M.D. Author info- Reusing images- Conflicts of interest:NoneMikael Häggström, M.D. - Own work, CC0, https://commons.wikimedia.org/w/index.php?curid=138436043; en.wikipedia.org/wiki/Colitis#/media/File:Histopathology_of_colonic_ulceration.jpg. This file is made available under the Creative Commons CC0 1.0 Universal Public Domain Dedication. No changes were made to this image).

(Figure 18 Crypt abscesses (luminal neutrophilic aggregates) in colitis)

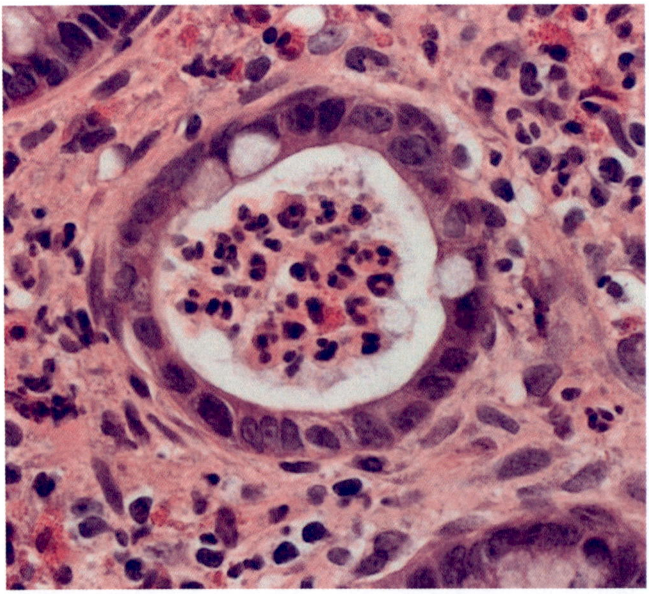

(This image is by Mikael Häggström, M.D. - Own work, CC0, https://commons.wikimedia.org/w/index.php?curid=125141216; en.wikipedia.org/wiki/Colitis#/media/File:Histopathology_of_a_crypt_abscess.jpg. This file is made available under the Creative Commons CC0 1.0 Universal Public Domain Dedication. No changes were made to this image).

(Immune-mediated endocrinopathies)

(The patterns of endocrinopathies differ between the inhibitors of the cytotoxic T-lymphocyte antigen 4 and programmed cell death protein 1 or programmed cell death protein 1 ligand pathways, but most often involve the thyroid and pituitary glands. The less common but important presentations include insulin-deficient diabetes mellitus, primary adrenal insufficiency, primary hypoparathyroidism, central diabetes insipidus, primary hypogonadism, and pancreatitis, with or without subsequent progression to diabetes mellitus or exocrine insufficiency).

(Thyroiditis causing both hyperthyroidism and hypothyroidism

Thyroid dysfunction is the most common endocrine immune-related adverse event associated with immune check point inhibitor therapy. Dysfunction can be in the form of either thyrotoxicosis or hypothyroidism, but the latter is the more common presentation. Thyrotoxicosis as the primary presentation is predominantly related to silent or destructive thyroiditis, and in most of these cases, hypothyroidism ensues shortly thereafter (median time 42 days).

(In some types of thyroiditis, physical examination may reveal an enlarged thyroid and/or tenderness to palpation. Hyperthyroid symptoms and signs vary between people and nervousness, irritability, increased perspiration, heart racing, hand tremors, anxiety, trouble sleeping, thinning of the skin, fine brittle hair, and muscular weakness - especially in the upper arms and thighs. More frequent bowel movements may occur, and diarrhea is common.

Common hypothyroid symptoms include poor ability to tolerate cold, fatigue, weight gain, feeling fuzzy -headed, depression, dry skin, and constipation).

(Figure 19. Symptoms and signs of hypothyroidism)

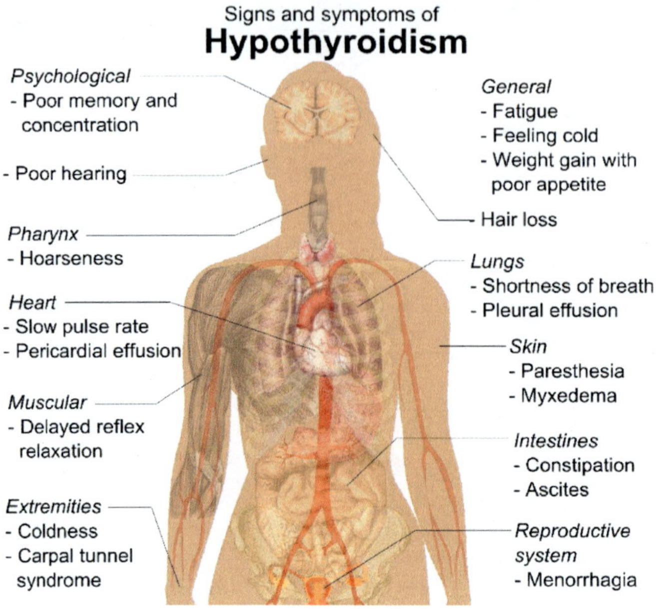

(This image is by Mikael Häggström. https://commons.wikimedia.org/w/index.php?curid=30556160; https://en.wikipedia.org/wiki/Hypothyroidism#/media/File:Signs_and_symptoms_of_hypothyroidism.png. This file is made available under the Creative Commons CC0 1.0 Universal Public Domain Dedication. No changes were made to this image).

(A meta-analysis of thyroid abnormalities due to check point inhibitor treatment in 38 randomized controlled trials calculated the overall incidence of hypothyroidism to be 6.6% (95% confidence interaval 5.5%–7.8%) and the incidence of thyrotoxicosis to be 2.9% (95% confidence interval 2.4%–3.7%.

With regard to severity, most of the thyroid-related adverse events are either asymptomatic (subclinical) or cause mild or moderate symptoms (CTCAE grade 1 or 2), with less than 1% leading to severe symptoms, hospitalization, or death (CTCAE grade 3 or higher.

The time of onset of thyroid dysfunction varies greatly, within the first 15 weeks of therapy in most reported cases, but as early as 7 days or as late as 3 years in others. Also, the time to onset is shorter with combined immunotherapy than with monotherapy).

(Hypophisitis)

(Figure 20. Anatomy of the pituitary gland)

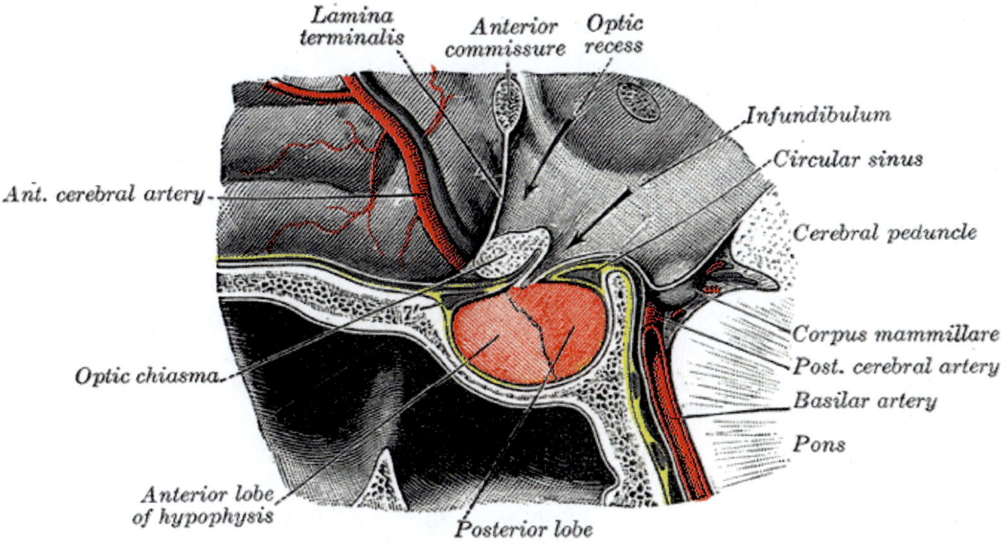

(This image is by Henry Vandyke Carter - Henry Gray (1918) Anatomy of the Human Body (See "Book" section below)Bartleby.com: Gray's Anatomy, Plate 1180, Public Domain, https://commons.wikimedia.org/w/index.php?curid=567162; https://en.wikipedia.org/wiki/Hypophysitis#/media/File:Gray1180.png. This work is in the public domain in its country of origin and other countries and areas where the copyright term is the author's life plus 100 years or fewer. This work is in the public domain in the United States because it was published (or registered with the U.S. Copyright Office) before January 1, 1929. No changes were made to this image).

(Immune check point inhibitor-induced hypophysitis affects the anterior pituitary [which secretes follicle-stimulating hormone, luteinizing hormone, adrenocorticotropic hormone, thyroid-stimulating hormone, prolactin, endorphins, and growth hormone], more often than it affects the posterior pituitary (which secretes antidiuretic hormone and oxytocin), and most patients have multiple hormonal deficiencies. One study of a meta-analysis reported that 36 (39%) of 92 patients on immune check point inhibitor regimens who developed hypophysitis had symptoms of grade 3 or higher on the Common Terminology Criteria for Adverse Events (CTCAE) scale).

(Central hypothyroidism is the most frequent complication, followed by hypogonadism. This is distinctive with the CTLA-4 inhibitor ipilimumab, suggesting that CTLA-4 is expressed preferentially by the thyrotropin-secreting and gonadotropin-secreting cells).

(Central adrenal insufficiency is also common and is concerning, as it can lead to life-threatening adrenal crisis.

Hypoprolactinemia: Prolactin levels are usually low; hyperprolactinemia is uncommon.

Growth hormone deficiency is rare, as the growth hormone axis is usually spared.

Diabetes insipidus is a very rare feature of hypopituitarism.

Immune check point inhibitor-induced hypophysitis-hypopituitarism is almost exclusively associated with the CTLA-4 inhibitor ipilimumab, and it appears to be the most common endocrinopathy associated with this drug, with incidences in the range of 10% to 15% reported. Cumulative dosage or cycle frequency do not appear to affect the incidence significantly.

However, the incidence is significantly higher with nivolumab-ipilimumab combination therapy (about 8%) than with ipilimumab alone (about 4%).

Hypophysitis-hypopituitarism occurs significantly less often with PD-1 inhibitors than with ipilimumab, and the presentations may drastically differ between the 2 drug classes, strongly suggesting independent pathways. Gland enlargement and combined axis dysfunction are more common in those treated with ipilimumab, whereas secondary adrenal insufficiency with subtle gland enlargement is more common with PD-1 inhibitors.

The median time of onset of hypophysitis-hypopituitarism is 8 to 10 weeks after initiating treatment, although this can vary by as much as 4 months.

Pituitary enlargement and hypophysitis usually resolve, but hypopituitarism can persist (with or without corticosteroidsteroid treatment) and may be permanent depending on the hormonal axis involved. The thyroid axis may recover in the long term, but recovery of corticotroph cell function is rare. Therefore, quality of life after immune check point inhibitor therapy poses a major issue for patients with secondary adrenal insufficiency).

(Pancreatic endocrine dysfunction: diabetes mellitus)

The adverse effects of immune check point inhibitor therapy on pancreatic endocrine function manifest in a similar manner to type 1 diabetes mellitus, with low or undetectable C-peptide and elevated autoantibody levels.

(Figure 21. Overview of the most significant symptoms of diabetes)

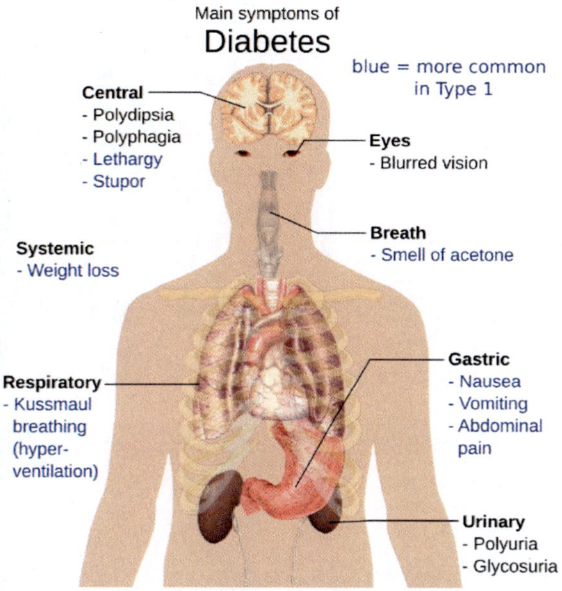

(This image is by Mikael Häggström, Public Domain, https://commons.wikimedia.org/w/index.php?curid=6055528; https://en.wikipedia.org/wiki/Diabetes#/media/File:Main_symptoms_of_diabetes.svg. The copyright holder of this work has released it into the publc domain. No changes were made to this image).

(Figure 22. Proliferative diabetic retinopathy, an advanced form of diabetic retinopathy, which occurs when abnormal new blood vessels and scar tissue form on the surface of the retina).

(This image is by http://www.nei.nih.gov/photo/eyedis/index.asp, Public Domain, https://commons.wikimedia.org/w/index.php?curid=862519; en.wikipedia.org/wiki/Diabetic_retinopathy#/media/File:Fundus_Proliferative_retinopathy_EDA01.JPG. This image is a work of the National Institutes of Health, part of the United States Department of Health and Human Services, taken or made as part of an employee's official duties. As a work of the U.S. federal government, the image is in the public domain. No changes were made to this image).

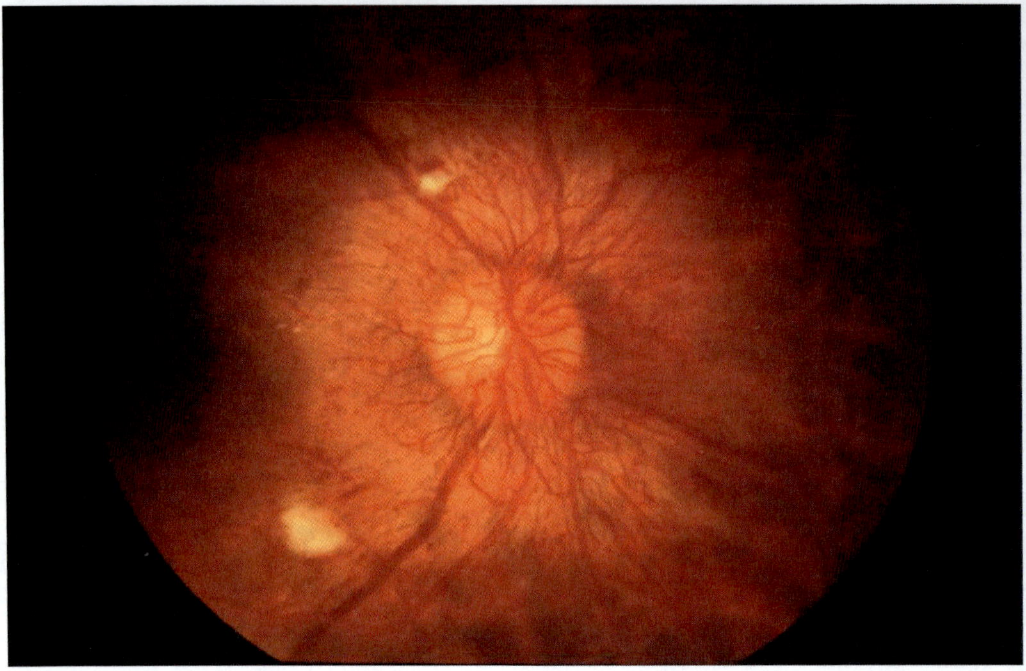

(Incidence rates have been reported to be between 0.2% and 0.9%, with 0.1% being CTCAE grade 3 or higher. However, there are recent reports of a more fulminant course with rapid-onset diabetic ketoacidosis associated with a disproportionately normal to mildly elevated hemoglobin A1c. Incidence rates are higher with PD-1 inhibitors (nivolumab, pembrolizumab), followed by PD-L1 inhibitors. Combination therapy may also increase risk, with a shorter onset of symptoms after initiation of therapy).

(One systematic review and meta-analysis of 71 cases reported that the mean age of the patients was 61.7 (± 12 years), 55% of cases were in men, and the median time to onset was 49 days (range 5–448 days) after starting check point inhibitor treatment. Half the patients had autoantibodies at presentation, with a higher incidence of diabetic ketoacidosis and more rapid onset of diabetes mellitus than in patients without autoantibodies. An at-risk DR or DQ allele was present in 85% of patients tested, similar to the rate in childhood-onset diabetes mellitus).

(Another systematic review reported comparable results, with similar incidences of diabetic ketoacidosis (71%) and islet autoantibodies (53%). However, fewer patients (65%) had susceptible HLA genotypes. These findings suggest a role of allele

screening in patients who may be at risk of immune check point inhibitor-induced diabetes).

(As in childhood-onset type 1 diabetes, lifelong insulin therapy is needed, and unlike other immune check point inhibitor endocrinopathies, pancreatic dysfunction does not respond to immunosuppressive therapy).

(Adrenal gland dysfunction)

(Immune check point inhibitor-associated primary adrenal insufficiency is an infrequent manifestation of immune-related adverse events.

(The adrenal cortex normally secretes glucocorticoids [primarily cortisol], mineralocorticoids [primarily aldosterone], and androgens. These hormones are important in regulating blood pressure, electrolytes, and metabolism as a whole. Deficiency of these hormones leads to symptoms ranging from abdominal pain, vomiting, muscle weakness and fatigue, low blood pressure, depression, mood and personality changes [in mild cases] to organ failure and shock [in severe cases]).

(Barroso-Sousa et al [3], in their meta-analysis and systematic review, reported only 43 cases of any grade primary adrenal insufficiency among 5,831 patients (0.7%), of which 14 (0.3%) were grade 3 or higher. In another study, among 256 patients who received ipilimumab, 2 cases of primary adrenal insufficiency (0.8%) were observed.

Another study reported that, of a total of 50,108 immune check point inhibitor-associated adverse events (reported using the World Health Organization's pharmacovigilance database of individual case safety reports over a decade), there were 451 cases of primary adrenal insufficiency, of which 45 were "definite" and 406 "possible." A small majority (51.8%) of the cases were in men, with a median age of 66 years. Most patients had received immune check point inhibitor monotherapy [nivolumab 44.3%, pembrolizumab 11.7%, and ipilimumab 23.6%], and 17.9% had received combination therapy. The median time to onset was 120 days [range 6–576]).

(Immune check point inhibitor-associated primary adrenal insufficiency is associated with significant rates of morbidity [> 90% of cases are severe] and mortality [7.3%].

(Mortality rates were similar in the subgroups receiving combination therapy vs monotherapy.

Melanoma recurrence may also be a concern, due to persistently elevated adrenocorticotropic hormone and melanocyte-stimulating hormone levels, although no studies to date have fully investigated this theory).

(Immune-mediated dermatologic reactions)

(Nonspecific immune activation by check point inhibitors may lead to immune-related adverse events, wherein the skin and its appendages are the most frequent targets [4]. Cutaneous immune-related adverse events include a diverse group of inflammatory reactions, with maculopapular rash, pruritus, psoriasiform and lichenoid eruptions being the most prevalent subtypes. Cutaneous immune-related adverse events occur early, with maculopapular rash presenting within the first 6 weeks after the initial immune check point inhibitor dose. Management involves the use of topical corticosteroids for mild to moderate [grades 1–2] rash, addition of systemic corticosteroids for severe [grade 3] rash, and discontinuation of immunotherapy with grade 4 rash. Bullous pemphigoid eruptions, vitiligo-like skin hypopigmentation/depigmentation, and psoriasiform rash are more often attributed to programmed cell death-1/programmed cell death ligand-1 inhibitors.

The treatment of bullous pemphigoid eruptions is similar to the treatment of maculopapular rash and lichenoid eruptions, with the addition of rituximab in grade 3–4 rash. Skin hypopigmentation/depigmentation does not require specific dermatologic treatment aside from photoprotective measures. In addition to topical corticosteroids, psoriasiform rash may be managed with vitamin D3 analogues, narrowband ultraviolet B light phototherapy, retinoids, or immunomodulatory biologic agents. Stevens-Johnson syndrome and other severe cutaneous immune-related adverse events, although rare, have also been associated with check pointblockade and require inpatient care as well as urgent dermatology consultation).

(Figure 23. Proriasis affecting the palms)

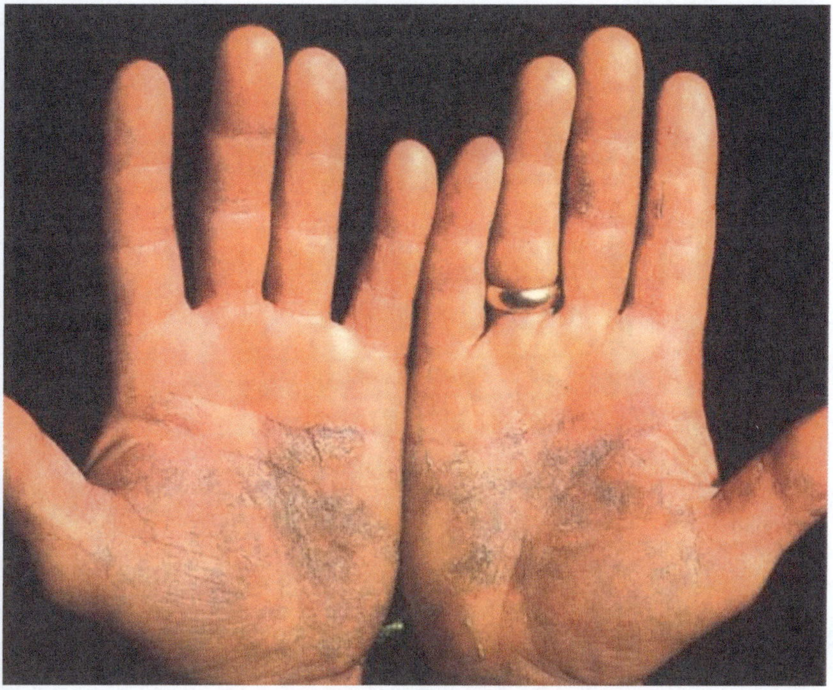

(This image is by US Military - http://history.amedd.army.mil/booksdocs/wwii/internalmedicinevolIII/chapter20figure100.jpg, Public Domain, https://commons.wikimedia.org/w/index.php?curid=1042690; https://en.wikipedia.org/wiki/Psoriasis#/media/File:Psoriasis_of_the_palms.jpg. This file is a work of a U.S. Army soldier or employee, taken or made as part of that person's official duties. As a work of the U.S. federal government, it is in the public domain in the United States. No changes were made to this image).

(Immune-mediated nephritis with renal dysfunction)

(Nephritis can produce glomerular injury, by disturbing the glomerular structure with inflammatory cell proliferation. This can lead to reduced glomerular blood flow, leading to reduced urine output and uremia. As a result, red blood cells may leak out of damaged glomeruli, causing hematuria.

Low renal blood flow activates the renin–angiotensin–aldosterone system, causing fluid retention and mild hypertension. As the kidneys become inflamed, they begin to excrete protein into the urine).

(Figure 24. The Renin–angiotensin-aldosterone system)

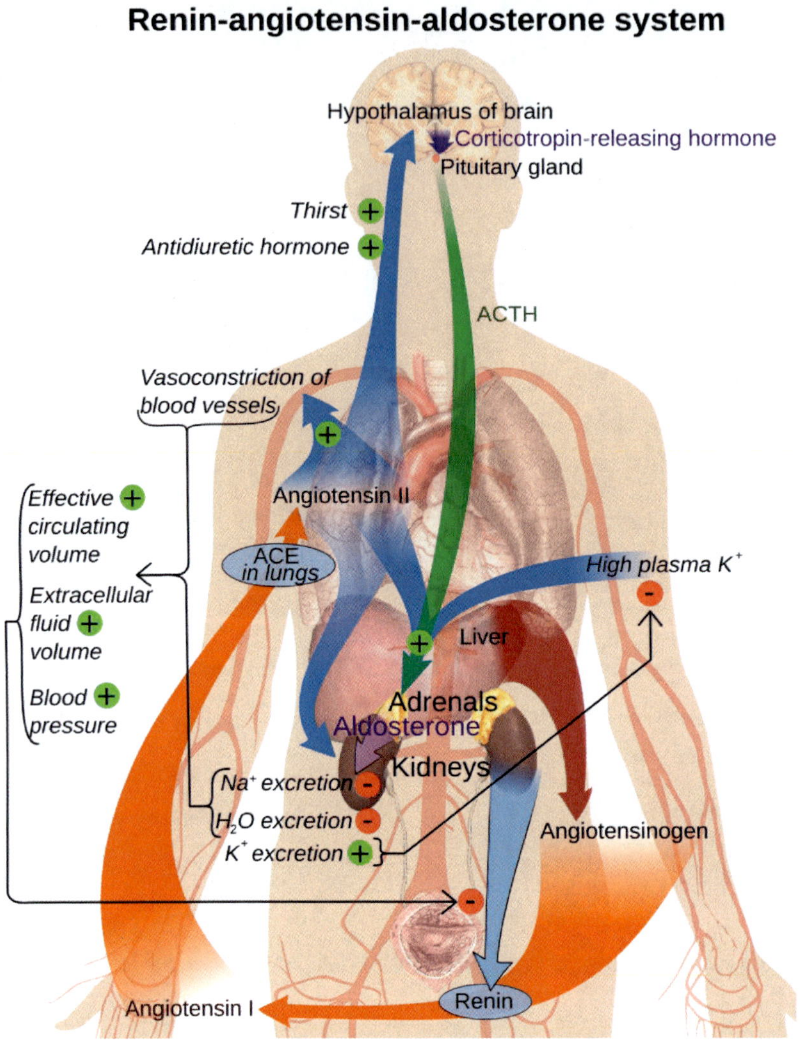

(This image is by Mikael Häggström, Public Domain, https://commons.wikimedia.org/w/index.php?curid=8458370; https://en.wikipedia.org/wiki/Nephritis#/media/File:Renin-angiotensin_system_in_man_shadow.svg. The copyright holder of this work has released this work into the public domain. No changes were made to this image).

(Immune-mediated myocarditis

Check point inhibitor-related myocarditis is a complex disease that has similarities in presentation to many other acute cardiac syndromes [5]. This overlap, along with the relative novelty of the entity with only a preliminary understanding about the pathophysiological characteristics, makes this a difficult condition to diagnose and treat. In addition, Check point inhibitor-related myocarditis is uncommon, making it difficult to study in a randomized manner, with most guidance being available from case reports and small case series. It is necessary for both the oncologist and cardiologist to have a high suspicion for this CI-related cardiac toxicity. Studies evaluating multimodality imaging and invasive testing with endomyocardial biopsy will guide development of better diagnostic algorithms for this condition. Current treatment is largely based on glucocorticoids with a possible role for more targeted immune modulators, depending on the clinical course of individual patients).

(Figure 25. Lymphocytic myocarditis (white arrow points to a lymphocyte), showing myocyte necrosis (black arrow), seen as hypereosinophilic cytoplasm with loss of striations).

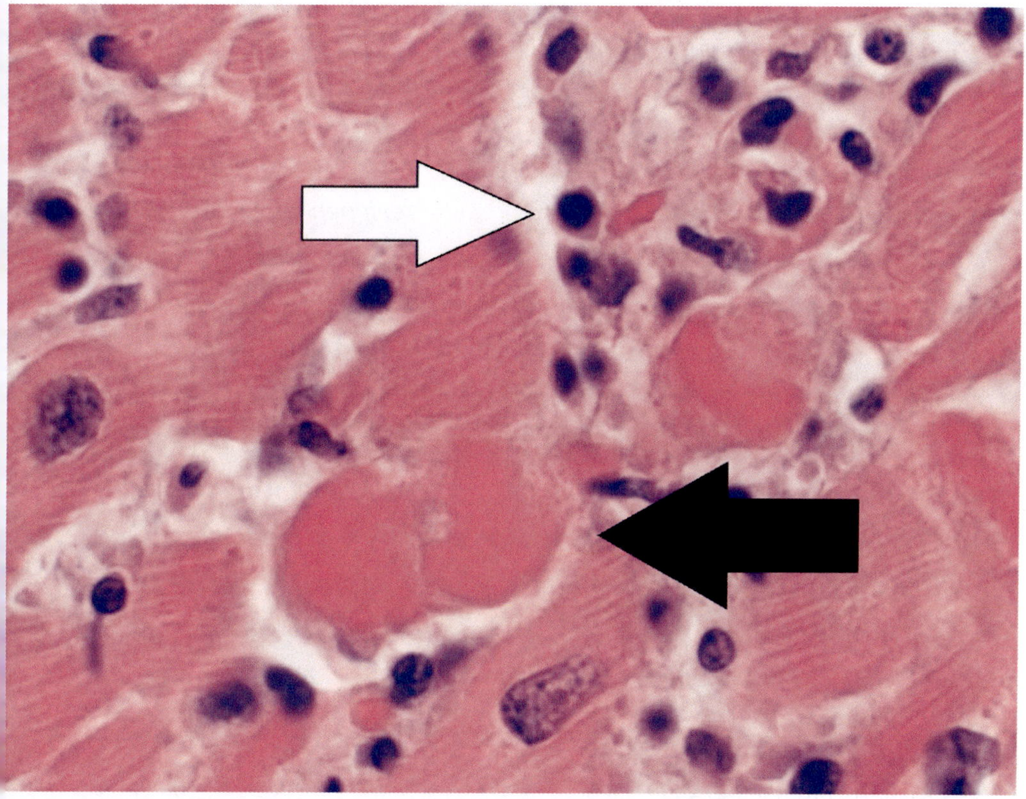

(This image is by Mikael Häggström, M.D. Own work, CC0, https://commons.wikimedia.org/w/index.php?curid=103645821; en.wikipedia.org/wiki/Myocarditis#/media/File:Histopathology_of_lymphocytic_myocarditis_with_myocyte_necrosis,_annotated.jpg. This file is made available under the Creative Commons CC0 1.0 Universal Public Domain Dedication. No changes were made to this image).

(There is wide variability in the reported time to onset of symptoms after starting CI treatment. In one study 35 patients with CI-associated myocarditis had a median

time of onset of 34 days (interquartile range, 21–75 days). In this cohort, 81% of patients presented within 3 months of initiating CI treatment, but late presentations of up to 454 days have been reported in the literature. Another study reported a range of 2 to 454 days and a median of 65 days to a diagnosis of cardiotoxicity after initiation of CI treatment. There was an average of 3 infusions administered before cardiotoxicity diagnosis.

Presentation can vary from asymptomatic elevations in cardiac biomarkers to severe decompensation with end-organ damage. The most concerning is the severe end of the spectrum manifesting as a fulminant or life-threatening presentation, in which patients present with a clinical syndrome of cardiogenic shock, and this may be accompanied by serious arrhythmias, such as advanced atrioventricular block or ventricular tachycardia. Patients can also present with concomitant pericardial effusion with or without pericarditis.

The two most common laboratory factors that may initially suggest the possibility of myocarditis are elevated serum troponin and natriuretic peptide levels. ECGs can help to identify myocarditis, although the findings are not specific. For patients receiving CI treatment, the possibility of myocarditis should be considered if any of the following are noted: new prolongation of the PR interval, atrioventricular block, ventricular arrhythmias, frequent premature ventricular complexes, ST depression, or diffuse T-wave inversions. Echocardiography is also an important tool to aid in the diagnosis of myocarditis, and to monitor the response to treatment. Of all the cardiovascular imaging modalities currently available, the one with the most robust validation to diagnose any myocarditis noninvasively at present is cardiovascular magnetic resonance. Endomyocardial biopsy is considered the gold standard diagnostic test for myocarditis.

The treatment of CI-associated myocarditis has largely been based on the use of glucocorticoids, including both oral prednisone and intravenous methylprednisolone).

ADVERSE REACTIONS

The most common adverse reactions (≥20%) are musculoskeletal pain, fatigue, rash, pruritus, and diarrhea. The most common laboratory abnormalities (≥20%) are decreased hemoglobin, decreased lymphocytes, increased AST, increased ALT, and decreased sodium.

To report SUSPECTED ADVERSE REACTIONS, contact Bristol-Myers Squibb at 1-800-721-5072 or FDA at 1-800-FDA-1088 or www.fda.gov/medwatch.

USE IN SPECIFIC POPULATIONS

• Lactation: advise not to breastfeed.

14. CLINICAL STUDIES

The efficacy of OPDUALAG was investigated in RELATIVITY-047 (NCT03470922), a randomized (1:1), double-blinded trial in 714 patients with previously untreated metastatic or unresectable Stage III or IV **melanoma**. Patients were allowed to have received prior adjuvant or neoadjuvant melanoma therapy: anti-PD-1, anti-CTLA-4, or BRAF-MEK inhibitors were allowed if received at least 6 months between the last dose of therapy and date of recurrence; interferon therapy was allowed if the last dose was at least 6 weeks prior to randomization. The trial excluded patients with active autoimmune disease, medical conditions requiring systemic treatment with moderate or high dose corticosteroids or immunosuppressive medications, uveal melanoma, and active or untreated brain or leptomeningeal metastases. Patients were randomized to receive OPDUALAG (nivolumab 480 mg and relatlimab 160 mg) by intravenous infusion every 4 weeks (n=355) or nivolumab 480 mg by intravenous infusion every 4 weeks (n=359) until disease progression or unacceptable toxicity. Randomization was stratified by tumor PD-L1 expression (≥1% vs.<1%) using PD-L1 IHC 28-8 pharmDx test, LAG-3 expression (<1% vs. >1%) using a clinical trial assay, BRAF V600 mutation status (V600 mutation positive vs. wild type), and M stage per the American Joint Committee on Cancer (AJCC) version 8 staging system (M0/M1 any[0] vs. M1 any [1]). The major efficacy outcome measure was progression-free survival (PFS) determined by Blinded Independent Central Review (BICR) using Response Evaluation Criteria in Solid Tumors (RECIST v1.1). Additional efficacy outcome measures were overall survival (OS) and overall response rate (ORR) determined by BICR using RECIST v1.1. Tumor assessments were conducted 12 weeks after randomization and continued every 8 weeks up to week 52 and then every 12 weeks. The trial population characteristics were: median age 63 years (range: 20 to 94); 58% male; 97% White 0.7% African American, and American Indian/Alaskan Native 0.1%; Hispanic 7%; and ECOG performance score was 0 (67%) or 1 (33%). Disease characteristics were: PD-L1 expression ≥1% (41%), LAG-

3 expression ≥1% (75%), AJCC Stage IV disease (92%), M1c disease (39%); M1d disease (2.4%), elevated LDH (36%), and BRAF V600 mutation-positive melanoma (39%).

The trial demonstrated a statistically significant improvement in PFS for patients randomized to the OPDUALAG arm compared with the nivolumab arm. The final analysis of OS was not statistically significant.

5.3. PEMBROLIZUMAB (KEYTRUDA)

KEYTRUDA® (pembrolizumab) injection, for intravenous use Initial U.S. Approval: 2014

INDICATIONS AND USAGE

KEYTRUDA is a programmed death receptor-1 (PD-1)-blocking antibody:

Melanoma

- for the treatment of patients with unresectable or metastatic melanoma.

(Figure 26. Gross pathology of a melanoma metastasis; the vast majority are pigment-forming, giving them a dark appearance).

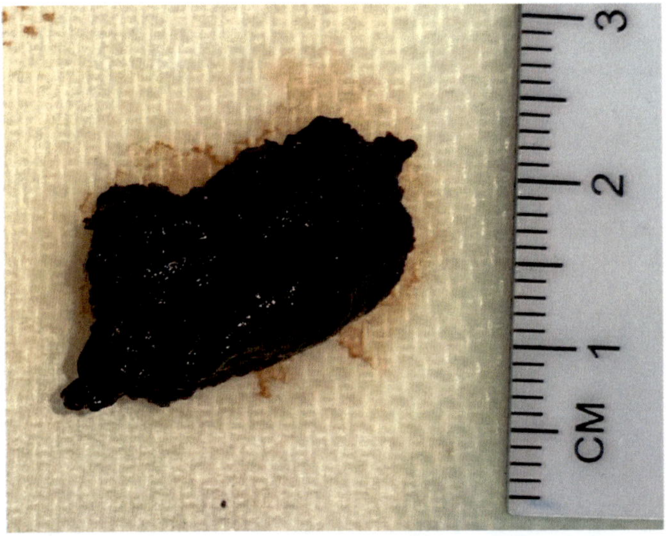

• for the adjuvant treatment of adult and pediatric (12 years and older) patients with Stage IIB, IIC, or III melanoma following complete resection

Non-Small Cell Lung Cancer (NSCLC)

• in combination with pemetrexed and platinum chemotherapy, as first-line treatment of patients with metastatic nonsquamous NSCLC, with no EGFR or ALK genomic tumor aberrations.

• in combination with carboplatin and either paclitaxel or paclitaxel protein-bound, as first-line treatment of patients with metastatic squamous NSCLC

• as a single agent for the first-line treatment of patients with NSCLC expressing PD-L1 [Tumor Proportion Score (TPS) ≥1%] as determined by an FDA-approved test, with no EGFR or ALK genomic tumor aberrations, and is:

o stage III where patients are not candidates for surgical resection or definitive chemoradiation, or o metastatic.

• as a single agent for the treatment of patients with metastatic NSCLC whose tumors express PD-L1 (TPS ≥1%) as determined by an FDA-approved test, with disease progression on or after platinum-containing chemotherapy. Patients with EGFR or ALK genomic tumor aberrations should have disease progression on FDA-approved therapy for these aberrations prior to receivinghttps://en.wikipedia.org/wiki/Melanoma#/media/File:Gross_pathology_of_melanoma_metastasis.jpg KEYTRUDA.

(Figure 27. Main sites of metastases for common cancer types. The included cancer types are the ones causing most death as per data from the USA in 2008. Lung cancer, mainly to adrenal glands, brain, and bone. Breast cancer, mainly to bone, liver, lung and brain. Colon cancer, mainly to liver. Pancreatic cancer, mainly to liver and lungs. Melanoma, mainly to brain. Ovarian cancer, mainly to pleural cavity and liver. Prostate cancer usually metastasizes to the bones [not shown in the diagram]).

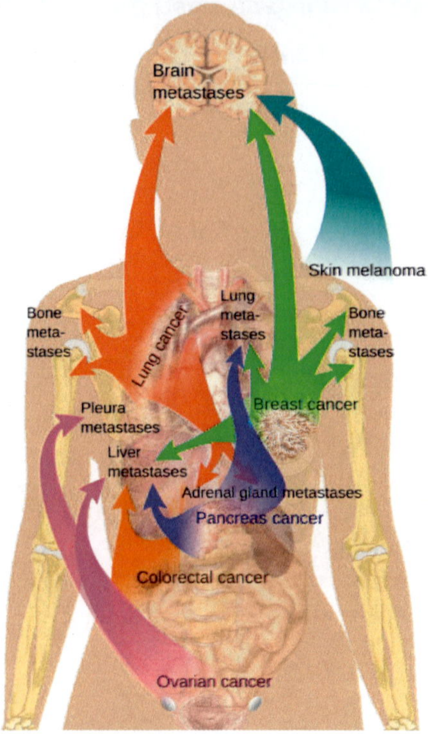

(This image is by Mikael Häggström - Image used is in the Public Domain, CC0, https://commons.wikimedia.org/w/index.php?curid=15275048; en.eikipedia.org.wiki/Metastsis#media/File: metastasis sites for common cancers.svg. This file is made available under the Creative Commons CC0 1.0 Universal Public Domain Dedication. No changes were made to this image).

Head and Neck Squamous Cell Cancer (HNSCC)

• in combination with platinum and FU for the first-line treatment of patients with metastatic or with unresectable, recurrent HNSCC.

• as a single agent for the first-line treatment of patients with metastatic or with unresectable, recurrent HNSCC whose tumors express PD-L1 [Combined Positive Score (CPS) ≥1] as determined by an FDA-approved test.

• as a single agent for the treatment of patients with recurrent or metastatic HNSCC with disease progression on or after platinum-containing chemotherapy

Classical Hodgkin Lymphoma (cHL)

• for the treatment of adult patients with relapsed or refractory cHL.

• for the treatment of pediatric patients with refractory cHL, or cHL that has relapsed after 2 or more lines of therapy.

(Figure 28. Photograph of Hodgkin's disease from a 1938 medical textbook, showing markedly enlarged left cervical lymph nodes).

(This image is by Unknown author - Scanned from Charles Phillips Emerson, Nellie Gates Brown, Essentials of medicine (J.B. Lippincott company, 1938), Public Domain, https://commons.wikimedia.org/w/index.php?curid=11291052; https://en.wikipedia.org/wiki/Hodgkin_lymphoma#/media/File:Hodgkin's_Disease_(Essentials_of_Medicine).jpg. This work is in the public domain in the United States because it was published in the United States between 1929 and 1977, inclusive, without a copyright notice. No changes were made to this image).

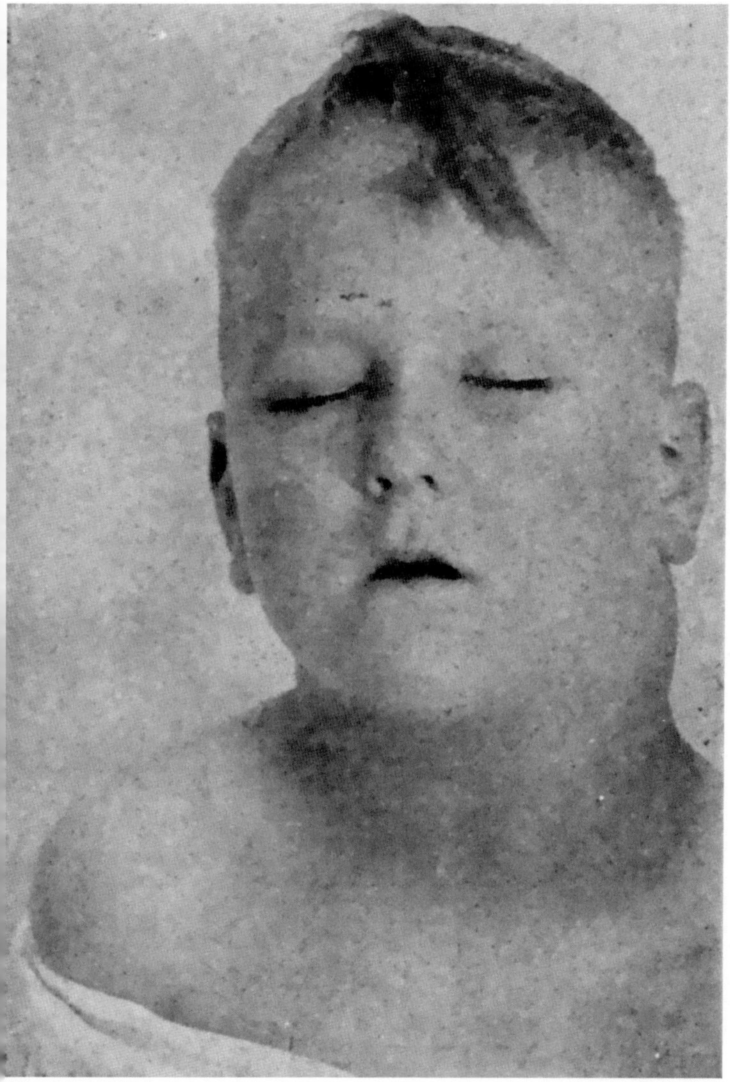

(*Figure 29. Photomicrograph of a classic Reed–Sternberg cell characteristic of Hodgkin Lymphoma*).

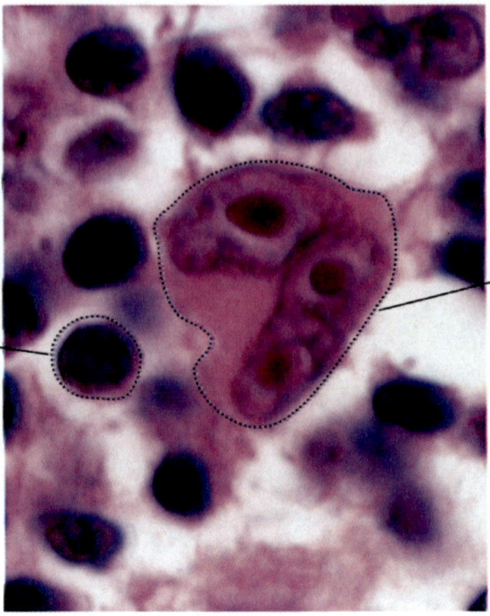

(This image is by Unknown author - National Cancer Institute, AV Number: CDR576466, Public Domain, https://commons.wikimedia.org/w/index.php?curid=5580965; en.wikipedia.org/wiki/Hodgkin_lymphoma#/media/File:Reed-Sternberg_lymphocyte_nci-vol-7172-300.jpg. This image is a work of the National Institutes of Health, part of the United States Department of Health and Human Services, taken or made as part of an employee's official duties. As a work of the U.S. federal government, the image is in the public domain. No changes were made to this image).

Primary Mediastinal Large B-Cell Lymphoma (PMBCL)

• for the treatment of adult and pediatric patients with refractory PMBCL, or who have relapsed after 2 or more prior lines of therapy. Limitations of Use: KEYTRUDA is not recommended for treatment of patients with PMBCL who require urgent cytoreductive therapy.

(Figure 30. Annotated version of Gray's image 969; opened Mediastinum viewed from left body side. In this disease the mass occurs in the anterior mediastinum).

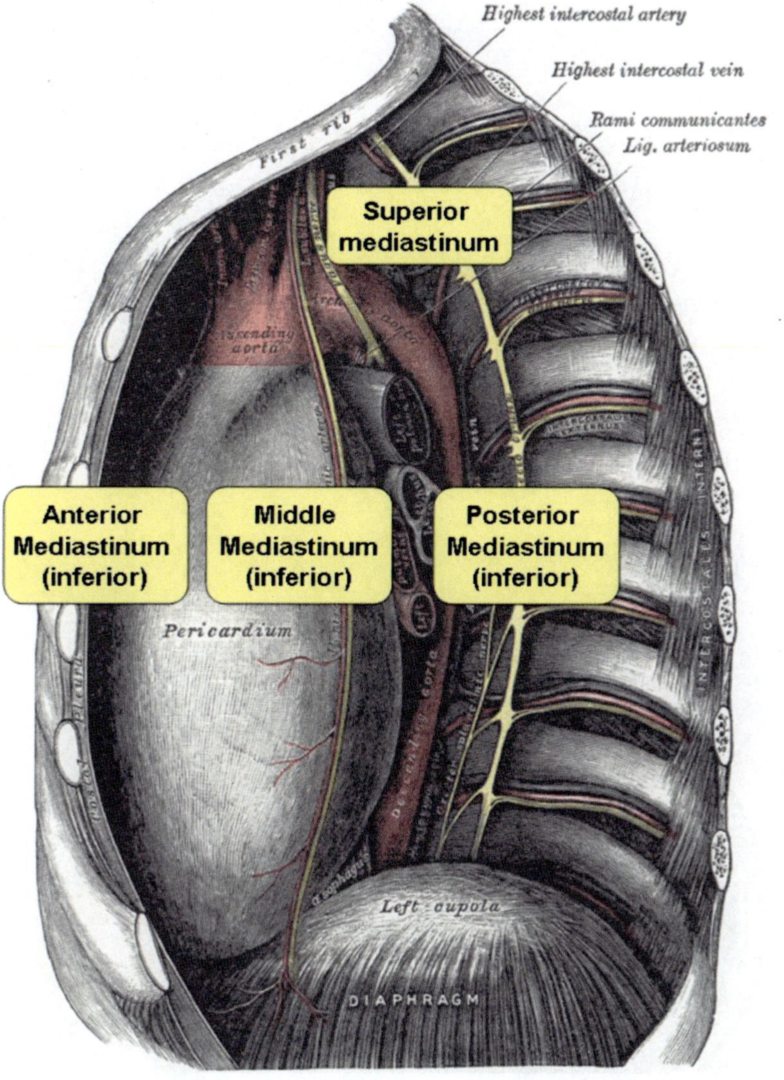

(This image is by No machine-readable author provided. Arcadian assumed (based on copyright claims). - No machine-readable source provided. Own work assumed (based on copyright claims)., Public Domain, https://commons.wikimedia.org/w/index.php?curid=1224440; en.wikipedia.org/wiki/Mediastinum#/media/File:Mediastinum.png. the copyright holder of this work, released this work into the public domain. No changes were made to this image).

Urothelial Carcinoma

• for the treatment of patients with locally advanced or metastatic urothelial carcinoma who:

o are not eligible for any platinum-containing chemotherapy, or

o who have disease progression during or following platinum-containing chemotherapy or within 12 months of neoadjuvant or adjuvant treatment with platinum containing chemotherapy.

• for the treatment of patients with Bacillus Calmette-Guerin (BCG)-unresponsive, high-risk, non-muscle invasive bladder cancer (NMIBC) with carcinoma in situ (CIS) with or without papillary tumors who are ineligible for or have elected not to undergo cystectomy.

(Figure 31. Bladder tumor on CT/PET scan. The uptake cranial to the lesion is physiological uptake in the colon).

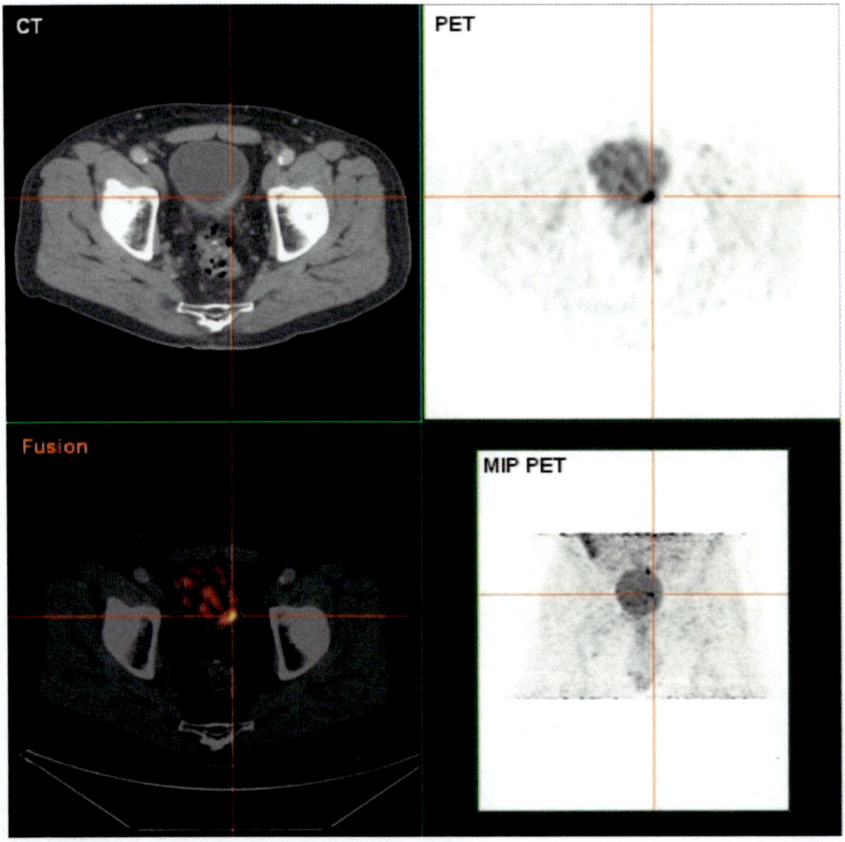

(This image is by Hg6996 - Own work, Public Domain, https://commons.wikimedia.org/w/index.php?curid=10765356; https://en.wikipedia.org/wiki/Bladder_cancer#/media/File:Blasentumor.jpg. The copyright holder of this work has released this work into the public domain. No changes were made to this image).

(Figure 32. Lymph nodes in the pelvis. Bladder cancer commonly spreads to obturator and internal iliac lymph nodes (not labelled in this image).

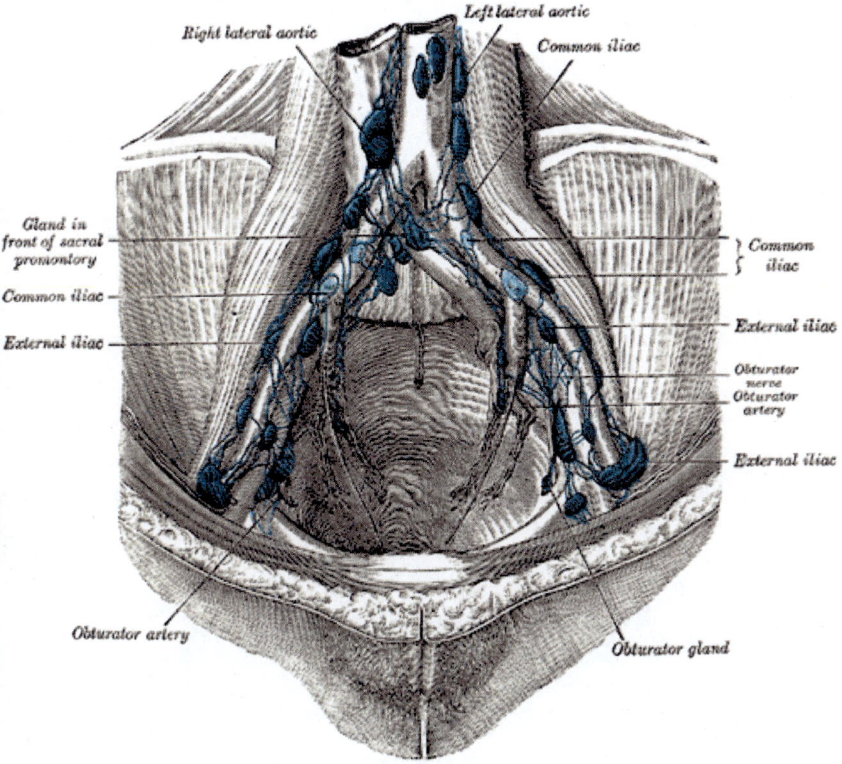

(This image is by Henry Vandyke Carter - Henry Gray (1918) Anatomy of the Human Body (See "Book" section below) Bartleby.com: Gray's Anatomy, Plate 611, Public Domain, https://commons.wikimedia.org/w/index.php?curid=566559, en.wikipedia.org/wiki/Bladder_cancer#/media/File:Gray611.png. This work is in the public domain in its country of origin and other countries and areas where the copyright term is the author's life plus 100 years or fewer. This work is in the public domain in the United States because it was published (or registered with the U.S. Copyright Office) before January 1, 1929. No changes were made to this image).

(Figure 33. Transitional cell carcinoma, being low-grade to the left, and high-grade to the right. H&E stain).

(This image is by Mikael Häggström, M.D. Own work, CC0, https://commons.wikimedia.org/w/index.php?curid=127894971 https://en.wikipedia.org/wiki/Transitional_cell_carcinoma#/media/File:Low-_and_high-grade_urothelial_carcinoma.jpg. This file is made available under the Creative Commons CC0 1.0 Universal Public Domain Dedication. No changes were made to this image).

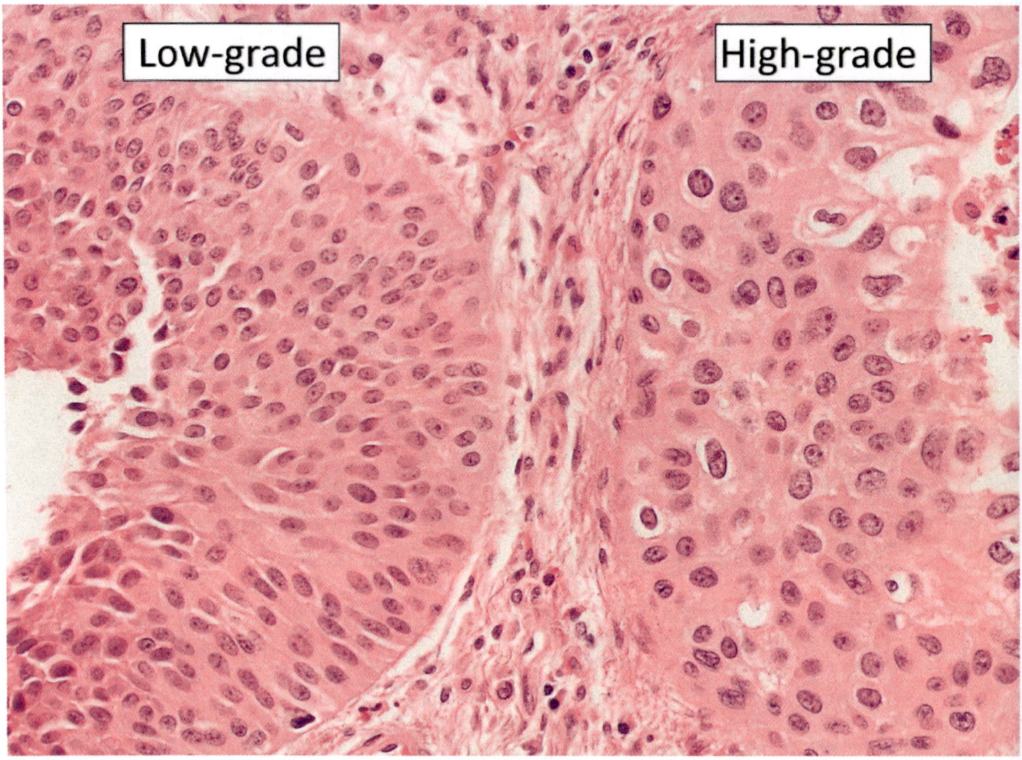

- **Microsatellite Instability-High or Mismatch Repair Deficient Cancer**

For the treatment of adult and pediatric patients with unresectable or metastatic, microsatellite instability-high (MSI-H) or mismatch repair deficient (dMMR) solid tumors that have progressed following prior treatment and who have no satisfactory alternative treatment options. Limitations of Use: The safety and effectiveness of KEYTRUDA in pediatric patients with MSI-H central nervous system cancers have not been established.

Microsatellite Instability-High or Mismatch Repair Deficient Colorectal Cancer (CRC)

For the treatment of patients with unresectable or metastatic MSI-H or dMMR colorectal cancer (CRC).

(Figure 34. Photomicrograph of colorectal adenocarcinoma, showing "dirty necrosis". Dirty necrosis consists of extensive central necrosis with granular eosinophilic karyorrhectic cell detritus. It is located within the glandular lumina, or often with a garland of cribriform glands in their vicinity).

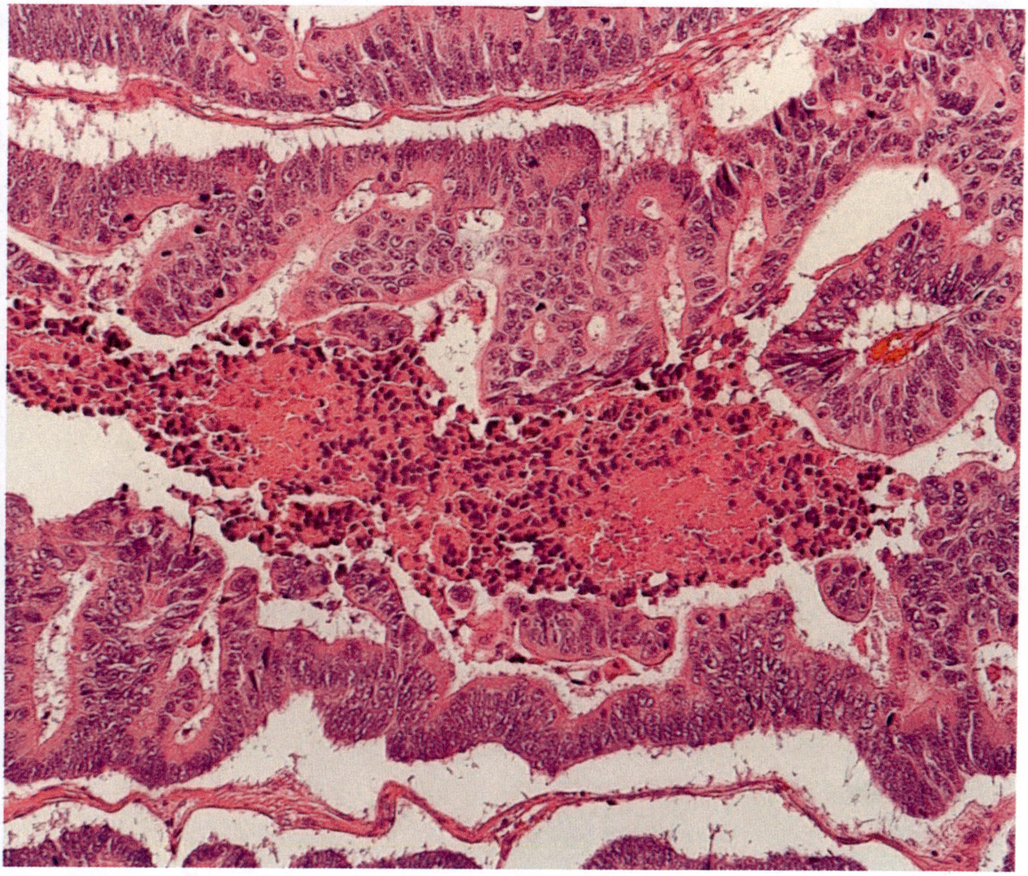

(This image is by Mikael Häggström, M.D. - Own work, CC0, https://commons.wikimedia.org/w/index.php?curid=83570643; Colorectal_cancer#/media/File:Micrograph_of_colorectal_carcinoma_with_dirty_necrosis.jpg. This file is made available under the Creative Commons CC0 1.0 Universal Public Domain Dedication. No changes were made to this image).

• **Gastric Cancer** in combination with trastuzumab, fluoropyrimidine-and platinum-containing chemotherapy, for the first-line treatment of patients with locally advanced unresectable or metastatic HER2-positive gastric or gastroesophageal junction (GEJ) adenocarcinoma.

(Figure 35. This cancer presented in a 40-year-old woman complaining of abdominal pain. Endoscopically it was a "very suspicious" ulcer. Biopsy showed diffusely infiltrating signet ring cell adenocarcinoma).

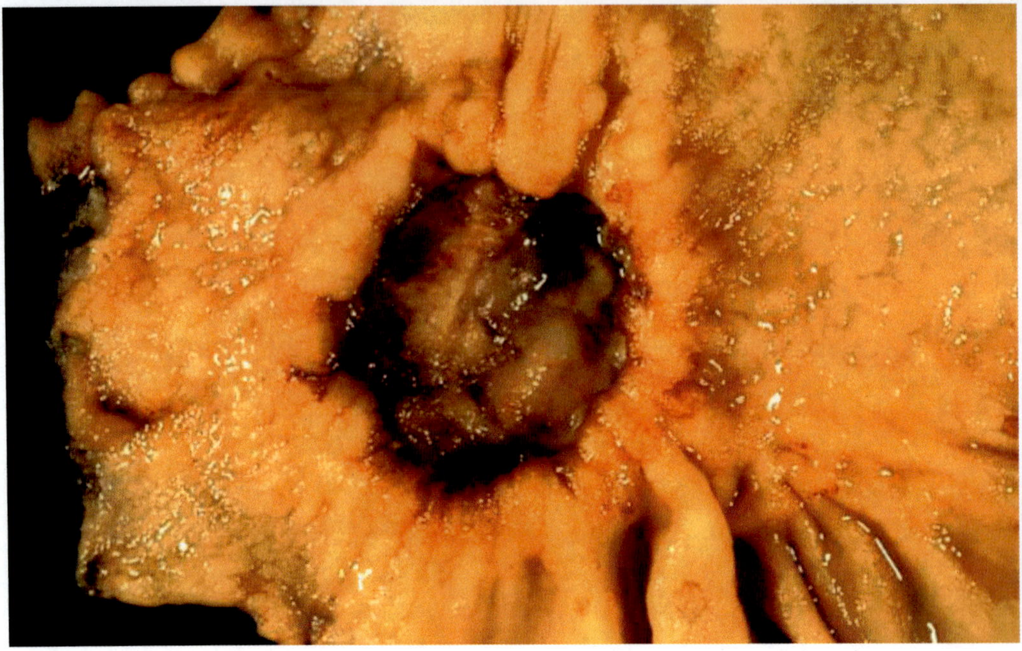

(This image is by http://web2.airmail.net/uthman/specimens/index.html, Public Domain, https://commons.wikimedia.org/w/index.php?curid=840055; en.wikipedia.org/wiki/Stomach_cancer#/media/File:Adenocarcinoma_of_the_stomach.jpg. This work has been released into the public domain by its author, Ed Uthman. This applies worldwide. No changes were made to this image).

• **Esophageal Cancer** for the treatment of patients with locally advanced or metastatic esophageal or gastroesophageal junction (GEJ) (tumors with epicenter 1 to 5 centimeters above the GEJ) carcinoma that is not amenable to surgical resection or definitive chemoradiation either:

o in combination with platinum-and fluoropyrimidine-based chemotherapy, or

o as a single agent after one or more prior lines of systemic therapy for patients with tumors of squamous cell histology that express PD-L1 (CPS ≥10) as determined by an FDA-approved test.

• **Cervical Cancer** in combination with chemotherapy, with or without bevacizumab, for the treatment of patients with persistent, recurrent, or metastatic cervical cancer whose tumors express PD-L1 (CPS ≥1) as determined by an FDA-approved test.

• as a single agent for the treatment of patients with recurrent or metastatic cervical cancer with disease progression on or after chemotherapy whose tumors express PD-L1 (CPS ≥1) as determined by an FDA-approved test.

• **Hepatocellular Carcinoma (HCC)** for the treatment of patients with HCC who have been previously treated with sorafenib.

(Figure 36. Primary liver tumor types by relative incidence in adults in the United States, with hepatocellular carcinoma at the left).

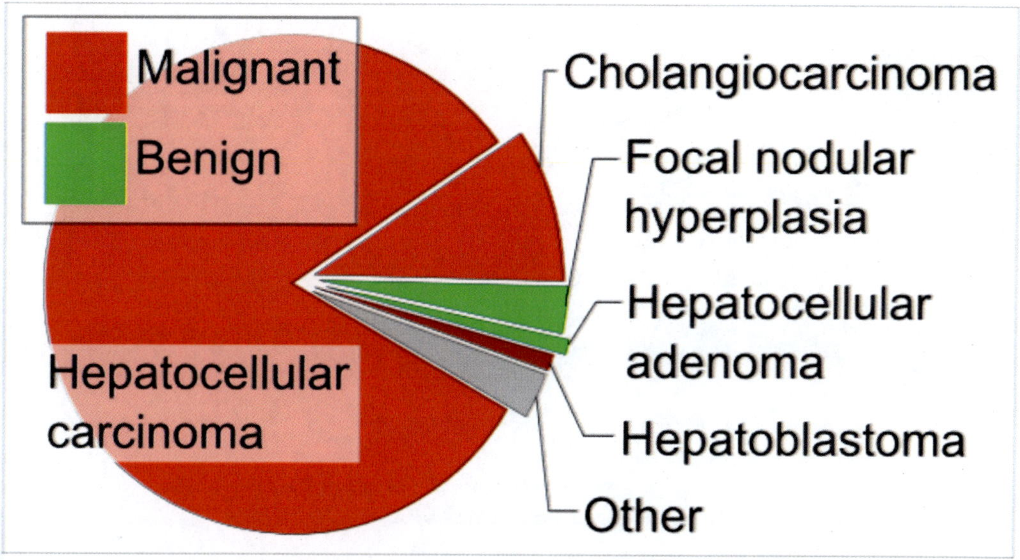

(This image is by By Mikael Häggström, M.D. Author info- Reusing images- Conflicts of interest:NoneMikael Häggström, M.D. - Own work, CC0, https://commons.wikimedia.org/w/index.php?curid=87423292; en.wikipedia.org/wiki/Hepatocellular_carcinoma#/media/File:Liver_tumor_types_in_adults_by_relative_incidence.png. This file is made available under the Creative Commons CC0 1.0 Universal Public Domain Dedication. No changes were made to this image).

(*Figure 37. Hepatocellular carcinoma This specimen is from a 50ish year old woman who presented to the hospital with abdominal pain and ascites. The radiologist recovered what appeared to be whole blood on paracentesis. Cytological exam of the bloody fluid showed no evidence of malignancy. Liver function tests were abnormal, and serologic tests were positive for antibody to hepatitis C. The patient deteriorated rapidly and died within a few days. The autopsy showed this hepatocellular carcinoma occupying much of the volume of a cirrhotic liver. Furthermore, the tumor had invaded the diaphragm and ruptured into the peritoneal cavity, causing the bloody ascites. The photo shows a view of a longitudinal slice taken through the full length of the liver).*

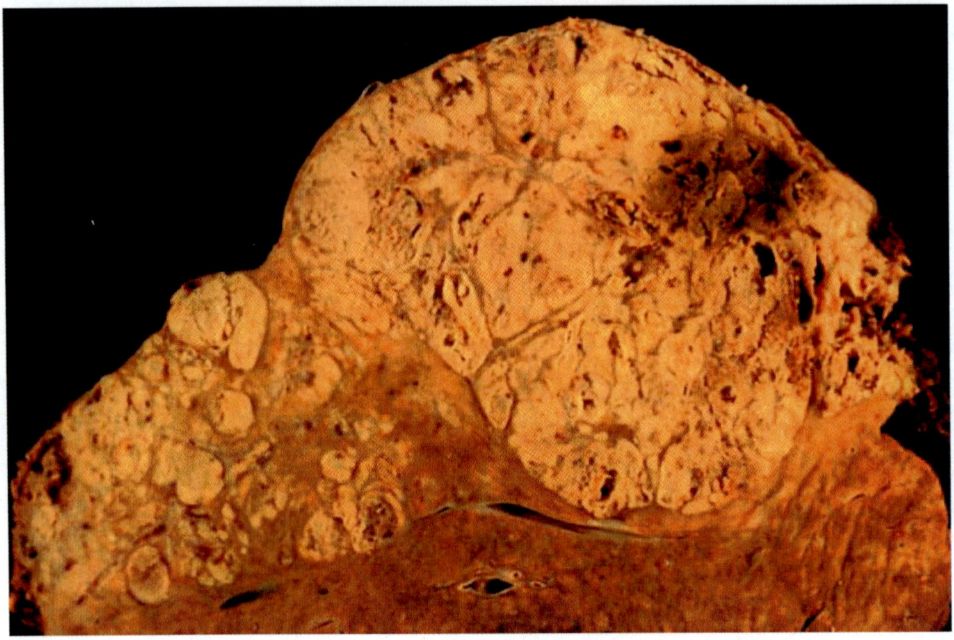

(This image is by http://web2.airmail.net/uthman/specimens/index.html, Public Domain, https://commons.wikimedia.org/w/index.php?curid=841059; en.wikipedia.org/wiki/Hepatocellular_carcinoma#/media/File:Hepatocellular_carcinoma_1.jpg. This work has been released into the public domain by its author, Ed Uthman. No change were made to this image).

- **Merkel Cell Carcinoma (MCC)** for the treatment of adult and pediatric patients with recurrent locally advanced or metastatic Merkel cellcarcinoma.

- **Renal Cell Carcinoma (RCC)** in combination with axitinib, for the first-line treatment of adult patients with advanced RCC.

- in combination with lenvatinib, for the first-line treatment of adult patients with advanced RCC.

- for the adjuvant treatment of patients with RCC at intermediate-high or high risk of recurrence following nephrectomy, or following nephrectomy and resection of metastatic lesions.

(Figure 38. Renal cell carcinoma).

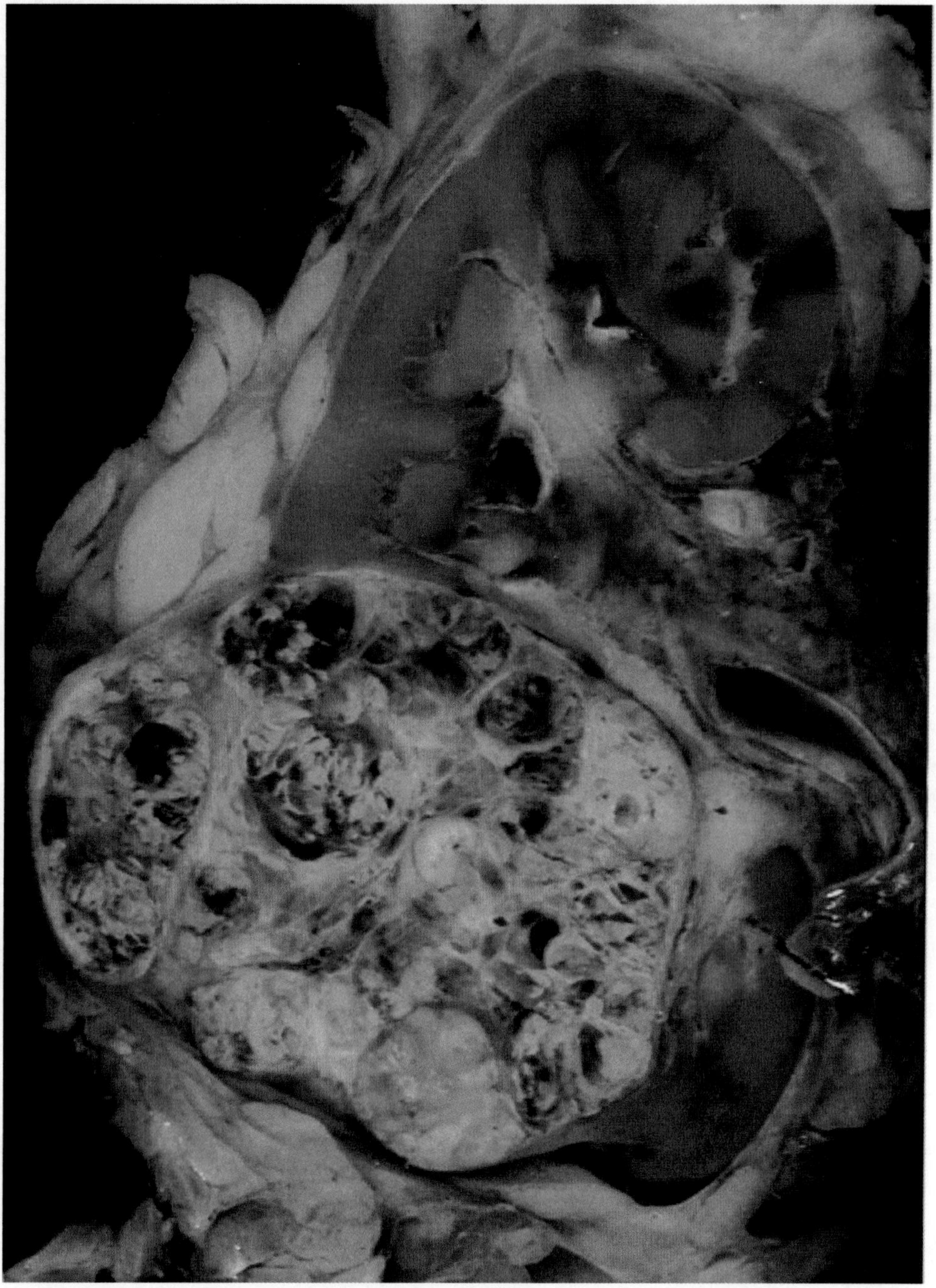

(This image is by Ed Uthman, MD (1953–) - http://web2.airmail.net/uthman/specimens/images/renal_cell_ca.html, Public Domain, https://commons.wikimedia.org/w/index.php?curid=841054; en.wikipedia.org/wiki/Renal_cell_carcinoma#/media/File:Renal_cell_carcinoma.jpg. This work has been released into the public domain by its author, Ed Uthman. No changes were made to this image).

• **Endometrial Carcinoma** in combination with lenvatinib, for the treatment of patients with advanced endometrial carcinoma that is not MSI-H or dMMR, who have disease progression following prior systemic therapy in any setting and are not candidates for curative surgery or radiation.

(Figure 39. Vaginal ultrasonography with an endometrial fluid accumulation (darker area) in a postmenopausal uterus, a finding that is highly suspicious for endometrial cancer).

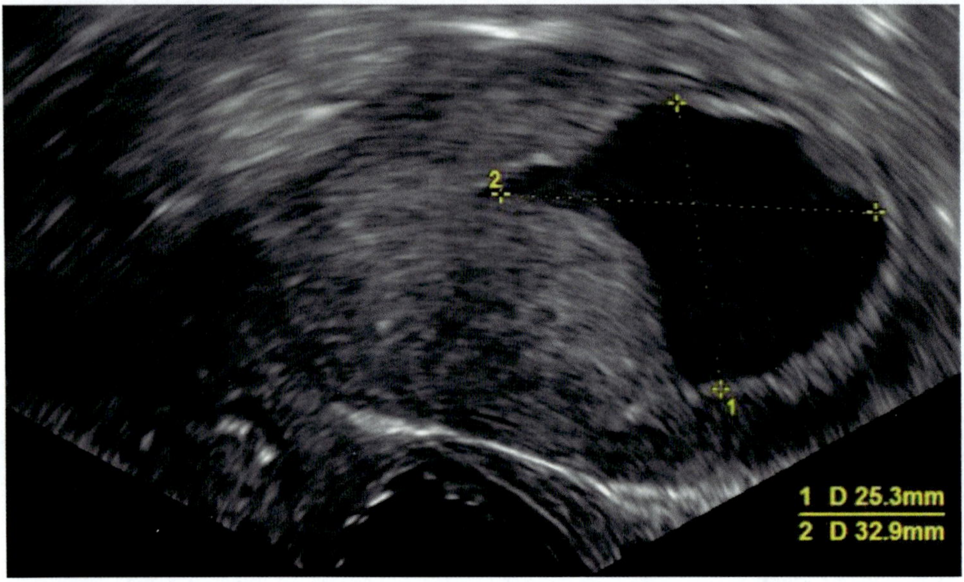

(Figure 40. Endometrial carcinoma.

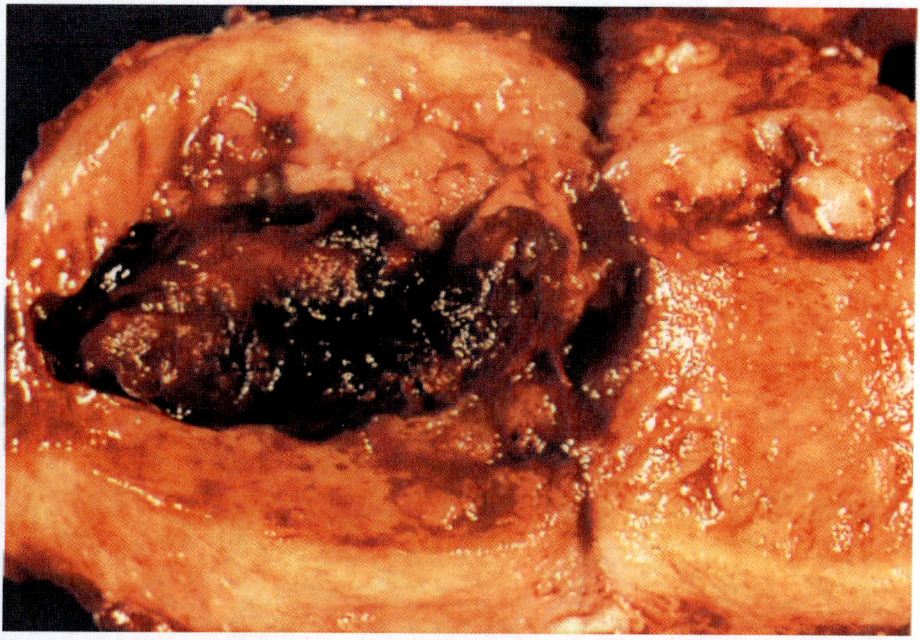

(This image was obtained from the Pathology Information Educational Resource (PEIR) website (http://peir.net/) PEIR Image# 402565. This work is in the public domain in the United States because it is a work prepared by an officer or employee of the United States Government as part of that person's official duties under the terms of Title 17, Chapter 1, Section 105 of the US Code).

• **Tumor Mutational Burden-High (TMB-H) Cancer** for the treatment of adult and pediatric patients with unresectable or metastatic tumor mutational burden-high (TMB-H) [≥10 mutations/megabase (mut/Mb)] solid tumors, as determined by an FDA-approved test, that have progressed following prior treatment and who have no satisfactory alternative treatment options. Limitations of Use: The safety and effectiveness of KEYTRUDA in pediatric patients with TMB-H central nervous system cancers have not been established.

• **Cutaneous Squamous Cell Carcinoma (cSCC)** for the treatment of patients with recurrent or metastatic cSCC or locally advanced cSCC that is not curable by surgery or radiation.

(Figure 41. Squamous Cell Carcinoma of the Skin. Tends to arise from pre-malignant lesions, actinic keratoses; surface is usually scaley and often ulcerates).

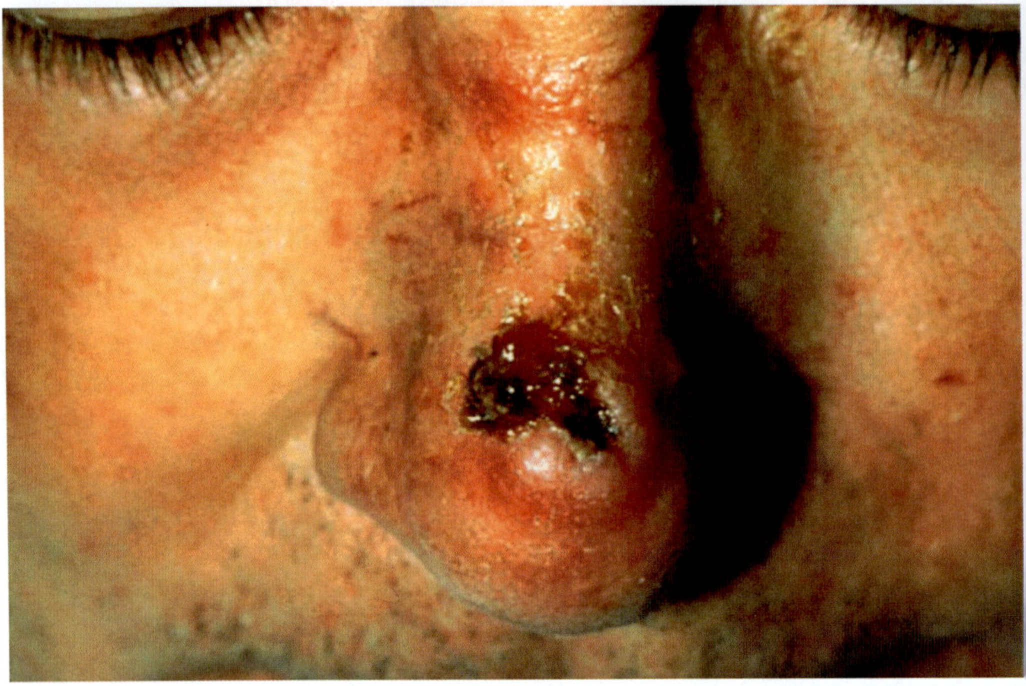

(This image is by Unknown photographer/artist - http://visualsonline.cancer.gov/details.cfm?imageid=2165, Public Domain, https://commons.wikimedia.org/w/index.php?curid=859316; en.wikipedia.org/wiki/Cutaneous_squamous-cell_carcinoma#/media/File:Squamous_Cell_Carcinoma.jpg. This work is in the public domain in the United States because it is a work prepared by an officer or employee of the United States Government as part of that person's official duties under the terms of Title 17, Chapter 1, Section 105 of the US Code. No changes were made to this image).

Figure 42. Histopathology of squamous-cell carcinoma in situ (black arrow), compared to normal skin on the right side of the photograph, showing marked atypia.

(This image is by Mikael Häggström, M.D. - Own work, CC0, https://commons.wikimedia.org/w/index.php?curid=85777987; en.wikipedia.org/wiki/Cutaneous_squamous-cell_carcinoma#/media/File:Histopathology_of_squamous_cell_carcinoma_in_situ.jpg. This file is made available under the Creative Commons CC0 1.0 Universal Public Domain Dedication. No changes were made to this image).

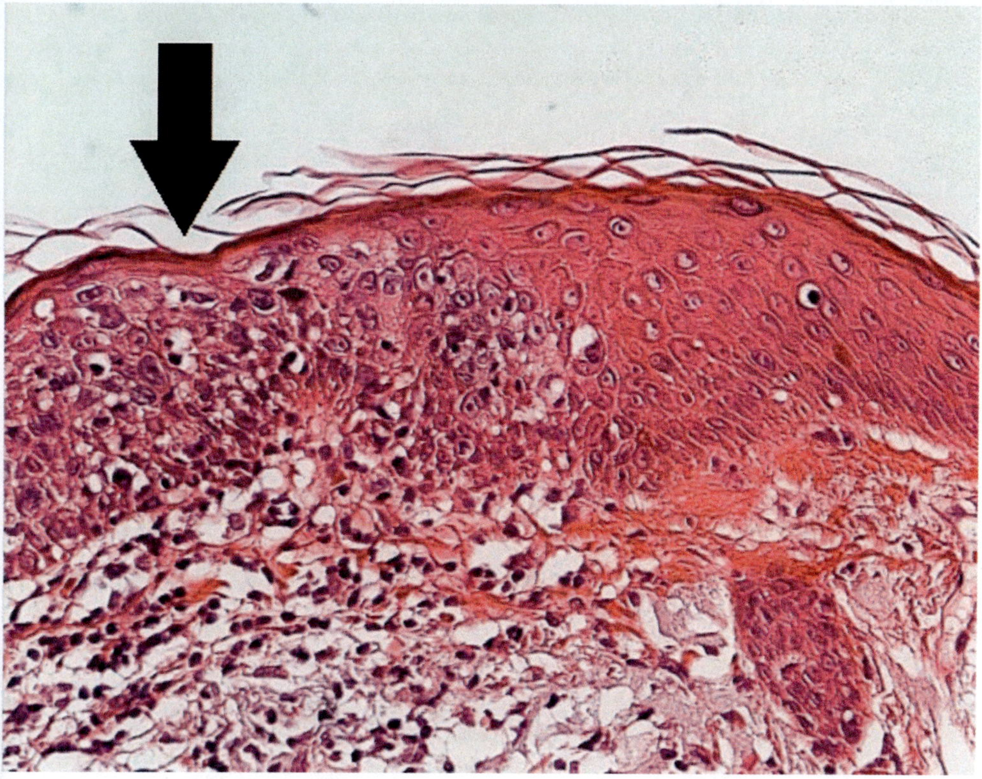

(Figure 43. Gross slice of squamous-cell carcinoma of the skin)

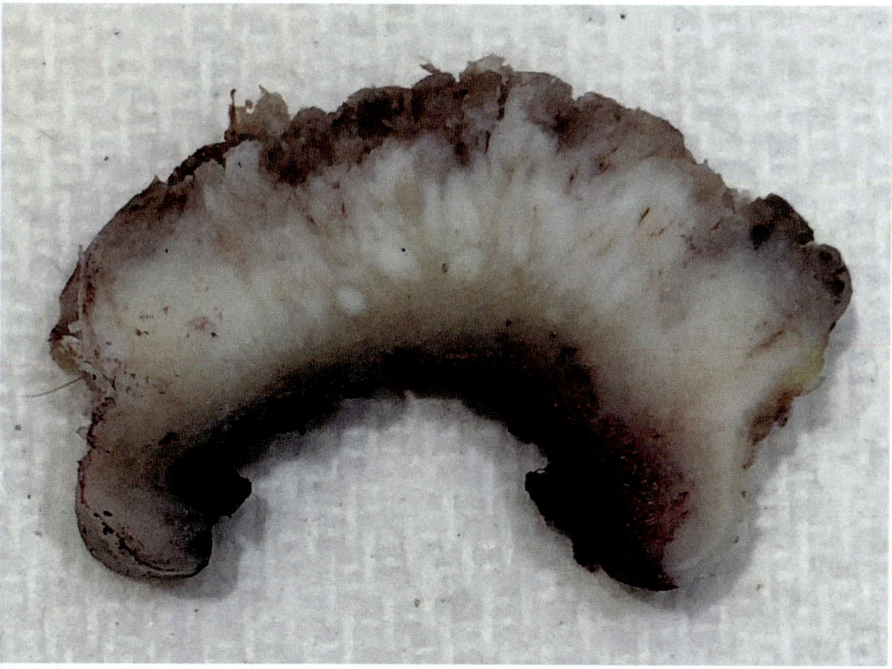

(This image is by Mikael Häggström, M.D - Own work, CC0, https://commons.wikimedia.org/w/index.php?curid=96668633; en.wikipedia.org/wiki/Cutaneous_squamous-cell_carcinoma#/media/File:Gross_pathology_of_squamous_cell_carcinoma.jpg. This file is made available under the Creative Commons CC0 1.0 Universal Public Domain Dedication. No changes were made to this image).

- **Triple-Negative Breast Cancer (TNBC)** for the treatment of patients with high-risk early-stage TNBC in combination with chemotherapy as neoadjuvant treatment, and then continued as a single agent as adjuvant treatment after surgery.

- In combination with chemotherapy, for the treatment of patients with locally recurrent unresectable or metastatic TNBC whose tumors express PD-L1 (CPS ≥10) as determined by an FDA approved test.

Adult indications: additional dosing regimen of 400 mg every 6 weeks for use at an additional recommended dosage of 400 mg every 6 weeks for all approved adult indications. This indication is approved under accelerated approval based on tumor response rate and durability of response. Continued approval for this indication may be contingent upon verification and description of clinical benefit in the confirmatory trials. This indication is approved under accelerated approval based on pharmacokinetic data, the relationship of exposure to efficacy, and the relationship of exposure to safety. Continued approval for this dosing may be contingent upon verification and description of clinical benefit in the confirmatory trials.

MECHANISM OF ACTION

Binding of the PD-1 ligands, PD-L1 and PD-L2, to the PD-1 receptor found on T cells, inhibits T cell proliferation and cytokine production. Upregulation of PD-1 ligands occurs in some tumors and signalling through this pathway can contribute to inhibition of active T-cell immune surveillance of tumors. Pembrolizumab is a monoclonal antibody that binds to the PD-1 receptor and blocks its interaction with PD-L1 and PD-L2, releasing PD-1 pathway-mediated inhibition of the immune response, including the anti-tumor immune response. In syngeneic mouse tumor models, blocking PD-1 activity resulted in decreased tumor growth.

WARNINGS AND PRECAUTIONS

Severe and Fatal Immune-Mediated Adverse Reactions

KEYTRUDA is a monoclonal antibody that belongs to a class of drugs that bind to either the programmed death-receptor 1 (PD-1) or the PD-ligand 1 (PD-L1), blocking the PD-1/PD-L1 pathway, thereby removing inhibition of the immune response, potentially breaking peripheral tolerance and inducing immune-mediated adverse reactions. Important immune-mediated adverse reactions listed under WARNINGS AND PRECAUTIONS may not include all possible severe and fatal immune-mediated adverse reactions. Immune-mediated adverse reactions, which may be severe or fatal, can occur in any organ system or tissue and can affect more than one body system simultaneously. Immune-mediated adverse reactions can occur at any time after starting treatment with a PD-1/PD-L1 blocking antibody. While immune-mediated adverse reactions usually manifest during treatment with PD-1/PD-L1 blocking antibodies, immune-mediated adverse reactions can also manifest after discontinuation of PD-1/PD-L1 blocking antibodies. Early identification and management of immune-mediated adverse reactions are essential to ensure safe use of PD-1/PD-L1 blocking antibodies. Monitor patients closely for symptoms and signs that may be clinical manifestations of underlying immune-mediated adverse reactions. Evaluate liver enzymes, creatinine, and thyroid function at baseline and periodically during treatment. In cases of suspected immune-mediated adverse reactions, initiate appropriate workup to exclude alternative etiologies, including infection. Institute medical management promptly, including specialty consultation as appropriate. Withhold or permanently discontinue KEYTRUDA depending on severity In general, if KEYTRUDA requires interruption or discontinuation, administer systemic corticosteroid therapy (1 to 2 mg/kg/day prednisone or equivalent) until improvement to Grade 1 or less. Upon improvement to Grade 1 or less, initiate corticosteroid taper and continue to taper over at least 1 month. Consider administration of other systemic immunosuppressants in patients whose immune-mediated adverse reactions are not controlled with corticosteroid therapy.

(Further clinical information on immune-mediated adverse reactions is given in the section on nivolumab).

14. CLINICAL STUDIES

14.1. MELANOMA

Ipilimumab-Naive Melanoma

The efficacy of KEYTRUDA was investigated in KEYNOTE-006 (NCT01866319), a randomized (1:1:1), open-label, multicenter, active-controlled trial in 834 patients. Patients were randomized to receive KEYTRUDA at a dose of 10 mg/kg intravenously every 2 weeks or 10 mg/kg intravenously every 3 weeks until disease progression or unacceptable toxicity or to ipilimumab 3 mg/kg intravenously every 3 weeks for 4 doses unless discontinued earlier for disease progression or unacceptable toxicity. Patients with disease progression could receive additional doses of treatment unless disease progression was symptomatic, was rapidly progressive, required urgent intervention, occurred with a decline in performance status, or was confirmed at 4 to 6 weeks with repeat imaging. Randomization was stratified by line of therapy (0 vs. 1), ECOG PS (0 vs. 1), and PD-L1 expression equal to, or greater than, 1% of tumor cells [positive] vs. <1% of tumor cells [negative] according to an investigational use only (IUO) assay. Key eligibility criteria were unresectable or metastatic melanoma; no prior ipilimumab; and no more than one prior systemic treatment for metastatic melanoma. Patients with BRAF V600E mutation-positive melanoma were not required to have received prior BRAF inhibitor therapy. Patients with autoimmune disease; a medical condition that required immunosuppression; previous severe hypersensitivity to other monoclonal antibodies; and HIV, hepatitis B or hepatitis C infection, were ineligible. Assessment of tumor status was performed at 12 weeks, then every 6 weeks through Week 48, followed by every 12 weeks thereafter. The major efficacy outcome measures were overall survival (OS) and progression-free survival (PFS; as assessed by blinded independent central review [BICR] using Response Evaluation Criteria in Solid Tumors [RECIST v1.1, modified to follow a maximum of 10 target lesions and a maximum of 5 target lesions per organ]). Additional efficacy outcome measures were objective response rate (ORR) and duration of response (DoR).

The study population characteristics were: median age of 62 years (range: 18 to 89); 60% male; 98% White; 66% had no prior systemic therapy for metastatic disease; 69% ECOG PS of 0; 80% had PD-L1 positive melanoma, 18% had PD-L1 negative melanoma, and 2% had unknown PD-L1 status using the IUO assay; 65% had M1c stage disease; 68% with normal LDH; 36% with reported BRAF mutation positive melanoma; and 9% with a history of brain metastases. Among patients with BRAF mutation positive melanoma, 139 (46%) were previously treated with a BRAF inhibitor.

The study demonstrated statistically significant improvements in OS and PFS for patients randomized to KEYTRUDA as compared to ipilimumab. Among the 91 patients randomized to KEYTRUDA 10 mg/kg every 3 weeks with an objective response, response durations ranged from 1.4+ to 8.1+ months. Among the 94 patients randomized to KEYTRUDA 10 mg/kg every 2 weeks with an objective response, response durations ranged from 1.4+ to 8.2 months.

Ipilimumab-Refractory Melanoma

The efficacy of KEYTRUDA was investigated in KEYNOTE-002 (NCT01704287), a multicenter, randomized (1:1:1), active-controlled trial in 540 patients randomized to receive one of two doses of KEYTRUDA in a blinded fashion or investigator's choice chemotherapy. The treatment arms consisted of KEYTRUDA 2 mg/kg or 10 mg/kg intravenously every 3 weeks or investigator's choice of any of the following chemotherapy regimens: dacarbazine 1000 mg/m2 intravenously every 3 weeks (26%), temozolomide 200 mg/m2 orally once daily for 5 days every 28 days (25%), carboplatin AUC 6 mg/mL/min intravenously plus paclitaxel 225 mg/m2 intravenously every 3 weeks for four cycles then carboplatin AUC of 5 mg/mL/min plus paclitaxel 175 mg/m2 every 3 weeks (25%), paclitaxel 175 mg/m2 intravenously every 3 weeks (16%), or carboplatin AUC 5 or 6 mg/mL/min intravenously every 3 weeks (8%). Randomization was stratified by ECOG PS (0 vs. 1), LDH levels (normal vs. elevated [≥110% ULN]) and BRAF V600 mutation status (wild-type [WT] or V600E). The trial included patients with unresectable or metastatic melanoma with progression of disease; refractory to two or more doses of ipilimumab (3 mg/kg or higher) and, if BRAF V600 mutation-positive, a BRAF or MEK inhibitor; and disease progression within 24 weeks following the last dose of ipilimumab. The trial excluded patients with uveal melanoma and active brain metastasis. Patients received KEYTRUDA until unacceptable toxicity; disease progression that was symptomatic, was rapidly progressive, required urgent intervention, occurred with a decline in performance status, or was confirmed at 4 to 6 weeks with repeat imaging; withdrawal of consent; or physician's decision to stop therapy for the patient. Assessment of tumor status was performed at 12 weeks after randomization, then every 6 weeks through week

48, followed by every 12 weeks thereafter. Patients on chemotherapy who experienced progression of disease were offered KEYTRUDA. The major efficacy outcomes were PFS as assessed by BICR per RECIST v1.1, modified to follow a maximum of 10 target lesions and a maximum of 5 target lesions per organ, and OS. Additional efficacy outcome measures were confirmed ORR as assessed by BICR per RECIST v1.1, modified to follow a maximum of 10 target lesions and a maximum of 5 target lesions per organ, and DoR. 78 Reference ID: 5425674 The study population characteristics were: median age of 62 years (range: 15 to 89), 43% age 65 or older; 61% male; 98% White; and 55% ECOG PS of 0 and 45% ECOG PS of 1. Twenty-three percent of patients were BRAF V600 mutation positive, 40% had elevated LDH at baseline, 82% had M1c disease, and 73% had two or more prior therapies for advanced or metastatic disease.

The study demonstrated a statistically significant improvement in PFS for patients randomized to KEYTRUDA as compared to control arm. There was no statistically significant difference between KEYTRUDA 2 mg/kg and chemotherapy or between KEYTRUDA 10 mg/kg and chemotherapy in the OS analysis in which 55% of the patients who had been randomized to receive chemotherapy had crossed over to receive KEYTRUDA. Among the 38 patients randomized to KEYTRUDA 2 mg/kg with an objective response, response durations ranged from 1.3+ to 11.5+ months. Among the 46 patients randomized to KEYTRUDA 10 mg/kg with an objective response, response durations ranged from 1.1+ to 11.1+ months.

Adjuvant Treatment of Resected Stage IIB or IIC Melanoma

The efficacy of KEYTRUDA was investigated in KEYNOTE-716 (NCT03553836), a multicenter, randomized (1:1), double-blind, placebo-controlled trial in patients with completely resected Stage IIB or IIC melanoma. Patients were randomized to KEYTRUDA 200 mg or the pediatric (≥12 years old) dose of KEYTRUDA 2 mg/kg intravenously (up to a maximum of 200 mg) every three weeks or placebo for up to one year until disease recurrence or unacceptable toxicity. Randomization was stratified by AJCC 8th edition T Stage (>2.0-4.0 mm with ulceration vs. >4.0 mm without ulceration vs. >4.0 mm with ulceration). Patients must not have been previously treated for melanoma beyond complete surgical resection for their melanoma prior to study entry. The major efficacy outcome measure was investigator-assessed recurrence-free survival (RFS) (defined as the time between the date of randomization and the date of first recurrence [local, in-transit or regional lymph nodes or distant recurrence] or death, whichever occurred first). New primary melanomas were excluded from the definition of RFS. Distant metastasis free survival (DMFS), defined as a spread of tumor to distant organs or distant lymph nodes, was an additional efficacy outcome measure. Patients underwent imaging every six months for one year from randomization, every 6 months from years 2 to 4, and then once in year 5 from randomization or until recurrence, whichever came first. The study population characteristics were: median age of 61 years (range: 16 to 87), 39% age 65 or older; 60% male; 98% White; and 93% ECOG PS of 0 and 7% ECOG PS of 1. Sixty-four percent had Stage IIB and 35% had Stage IIC.

The trial demonstrated a statistically significant improvement in RFS and DMFS for patients randomized to the KEYTRUDA arm compared with placebo.

Adjuvant Treatment of Stage III Resected Melanoma

The efficacy of KEYTRUDA was investigated in KEYNOTE-054 (NCT02362594), a multicenter, randomized (1:1), double-blind, placebo-controlled trial in patients with completely resected Stage IIIA (>1 mm lymph node metastasis), IIIB, or IIIC melanoma. Patients were randomized to KEYTRUDA 200 mg intravenously every three weeks or placebo for up to one year until disease recurrence or unacceptable toxicity. Randomization was stratified by the American Joint Committee on Cancer 7th edition (AJCC) stage (IIIA vs. IIIB vs. IIIC 1-3 positive lymph nodes vs. IIIC ≥4 positive lymph nodes) and geographic region (North America, European countries, Australia, and other countries as designated). Patients must have undergone lymph node dissection and, if indicated, radiotherapy within 13 weeks prior to starting treatment. The major efficacy outcome measure was investigator-assessed recurrence-free survival (RFS) in the whole population and in the population with PD-L1 positive tumors where RFS was defined as the time between the date of randomization and the date of first recurrence (local, regional, or distant metastasis) or death, whichever occurs first. New primary melanomas were excluded from the definition of RFS. DMFS in the whole population and in the population with PD-L1 positive tumors were additional efficacy outcome measures. DMFS was defined as a spread of tumor to distant organs or distant lymph nodes. Patients underwent imaging every 12 weeks after the first dose of KEYTRUDA for the first two years, then every 6 months from year 3 to 5, and then annually. The study population characteristics were: median age of 54 years (range: 19 to 88), 25% age 65 or older; 62% male; and 94% ECOG PS of 0 and 6% ECOG PS of 1. Sixteen percent had Stage IIIA, 46% had Stage IIIB, 18% had Stage IIIC (1-3 positive lymph nodes), and 20% had Stage IIIC (≥4 positive lymph nodes); 50% were BRAF V600 mutation positive and 44% were BRAF wild-type; and 84% had PD L1 positive melanoma with TPS ≥1% according to an IUO assay.

The trial demonstrated a statistically significant improvement in RFS and DMFS for patients randomized to the KEYTRUDA arm compared with placebo. For patients with PD-L1 positive tumors, the RFS HR was 0.54 (95% CI: 0.42, 0.69); p<0.0001. For patients with PD-L1 positive tumors, the DMFS HR was 0.61 (95% CI: 0.49, 0.76); p<0.0001. The RFS and DMFS benefit for KEYTRUDA compared to placebo was observed regardless of tumor PD-L1 expression.

14.2 NON-SMALL CELL LUNG CANCER

First-line treatment of metastatic non-squamous NSCLC with pemetrexed and platinum chemotherapy

The efficacy of KEYTRUDA in combination with pemetrexed and platinum chemotherapy was investigated in KEYNOTE-189 (NCT02578680), a randomized, multicenter, double-blind, active controlled trial conducted in 616 patients with metastatic non-squamous NSCLC, regardless of PD-L1 tumor expression status, who had not previously received systemic therapy for metastatic disease and in whom there were no EGFR or ALK genomic tumor aberrations. Patients with autoimmune disease that required systemic therapy within 2 years of treatment; a medical condition that required immunosuppression; or who had received more than 30 Gy of thoracic radiation within the prior 26 weeks were ineligible. Randomization was stratified by smoking status (never vs. former/current), choice of platinum (cisplatin vs. carboplatin), and tumor PD-L1 status (TPS <1% [negative] vs. TPS euqual or greater than 1% [positive].

Patients were randomized (2:1) to one of the following treatment arms: • KEYTRUDA 200 mg, pemetrexed 500 mg/m2, and investigator's choice of cisplatin 75 mg/m2 or carboplatin AUC 5 mg/mL/min intravenously on Day 1 of each 21-day cycle for 4 cycles followed by KEYTRUDA 200 mg and pemetrexed 500 mg/m2 intravenously every 3 weeks. KEYTRUDA was administered prior to chemotherapy on Day 1.

• Placebo, pemetrexed 500 mg/m2, and investigator's choice of cisplatin 75 mg/m2 or carboplatin AUC 5 mg/mL/min intravenously on Day 1 of each 21-day cycle for 4 cycles followed by placebo and pemetrexed 500 mg/m2 intravenously every 3 weeks.

Treatment with KEYTRUDA continued until RECIST v1.1 (modified to follow a maximum of 10 target lesions and a maximum of 5 target lesions per organ)-defined progression of disease as determined by the investigator, unacceptable toxicity, or a maximum of 24 months. Administration of KEYTRUDA was permitted beyond RECIST-defined disease progression if the patient was clinically stable and considered to be deriving clinical benefit by the investigator. Patients randomized to placebo and chemotherapy were offered KEYTRUDA as a single agent at the time of disease progression. Assessment of tumor status was performed at Week 6, Week 12, and then every 9 weeks thereafter. The main efficacy outcome measures were OS and PFS as assessed by BICR according to RECIST v1.1, modified to follow a maximum of 10 target lesions and a maximum of 5 target lesions per organ. Additional efficacy outcome measures were ORR and DoR, as assessed by BICR according to RECIST v1.1, modified to follow a maximum of 10 target lesions and a maximum of 5 target lesions per organ. The study population characteristics were: median age of 64 years (range: 34 to 84), 49% age 65 or older; 59% male; 94% White and 3% Asian; 56% ECOG PS of 1; and 18% with history of brain metastases. Thirty-one percent had tumor PD-L1 expression TPS<1% [negative]. Seventy-two percent received carboplatin and 12% were never smokers. A total of 85 patients in the placebo and chemotherapy arm received an anti-PD-1/PD-L1 monoclonal antibody at the time of disease progression.

The trial demonstrated a statistically significant improvement in OS and PFS for patients randomized to KEYTRUDA in combination with pemetrexed and platinum chemotherapy compared with placebo, pemetrexed, and platinum chemotherapy.

First-line treatment of metastatic squamous NSCLC with carboplatin and either paclitaxel or paclitaxel protein-bound chemotherapy

The efficacy of KEYTRUDA in combination with carboplatin and investigator's choice of either paclitaxel or paclitaxel protein-bound was investigated in KEYNOTE-407 (NCT02775435), a randomized, multi center, double-blind, placebo-controlled trial conducted in 559 patients with metastatic squamous NSCLC, regardless of PD-L1 tumor expression status, who had not previously received systemic therapy for metastatic disease. Patients with autoimmune disease that required systemic therapy within 2 years of treatment; a medical condition that required immunosuppression; or who had received more than 30 Gy of thoracic radiation within the prior 26 weeks were ineligible. Randomization was stratified by tumor PD-L1 status (TPS <1% [negative] or equal to, or greater than, 1% [positive], choice of paclitaxel or paclitaxel protein-bound, and geographic region (East Asia vs. non-East Asia). Patients were randomized (1:1) to one of the following treatment arms; all study medications were administered via intravenous infusion:

• KEYTRUDA 200 mg and carboplatin AUC 6 mg/mL/min on Day 1 of each 21-day cycle for 4 cycles, and paclitaxel 200 mg/m2 on Day 1 of each 21-day cycle for 4 cycles or paclitaxel protein-bound 100 mg/m2 on Days 1, 8 and 15 of each 21-day cycle for 4 cycles, followed by KEYTRUDA 200 mg every 3 weeks. KEYTRUDA was administered prior to chemotherapy on Day 1.

• Placebo and carboplatin AUC 6 mg/mL/min on Day 1 of each 21-day cycle for 4 cycles and paclitaxel 200 mg/m2 on Day 1 of each 21-day cycle for 4 cycles or paclitaxel protein-bound 100 mg/m2 on Days 1, 8 and 15 of each 21-day cycle for 4 cycles, followed by placebo every 3 weeks. Treatment with KEYTRUDA and chemotherapy or placebo and chemotherapy continued until RECIST v1.1 (modified to follow a maximum of 10 target lesions and a maximum of 5 target lesions per organ)-defined progression of disease as determined by BICR, unacceptable toxicity, or a maximum of 24 months.

Administration of KEYTRUDA was permitted beyond RECIST-defined disease progression if the patient was clinically stable and deriving clinical benefit as determined by the investigator. Patients randomized to the placebo and chemotherapy arm were offered KEYTRUDA as a single agent at the time of disease progression. Assessment of tumor status was performed every 6 weeks through Week 18, every 9 weeks through Week 45 and every 12 weeks thereafter. The main efficacy outcome measures were PFS and ORR as assessed by BICR using RECIST v1.1, modified to follow a maximum of 10 target lesions and a maximum of 5 target lesions per organ, and OS. An additional efficacy outcome measure was DoR as assessed by BICR according to RECIST v1.1, modified to follow a maximum of 10 target lesions and a maximum of 5 target lesions per organ. The study population characteristics were: median age of 65 years (range: 29 to 88), 55% age 65 or older; 81% male; 77% White; 71% ECOG PS of 1; and 8% with a history of brain metastases. Thirty-five percent had tumor PD-L1 expression TPS <1%; 19% were from the East Asian region; and 60% received paclitaxel.

The trial demonstrated a statistically significant improvement in OS, PFS and ORR in patients randomized to KEYTRUDA in combination with carboplatin and either paclitaxel or paclitaxel protein-bound chemotherapy compared with patients randomized to placebo with carboplatin and either paclitaxel or paclitaxel protein-bound chemotherapy.

First-line treatment of metastatic NSCLC as a single agent

The efficacy of KEYTRUDA was investigated in KEYNOTE-042 (NCT02220894), a randomized, multicenter, open-label, active-controlled trial conducted in 1274 patients with Stage III NSCLC who were not candidates for surgical resection or definitive chemoradiation, or patients with metastatic NSCLC. Only patients whose tumors expressed PD-L1 (TPS ≥1%) by an immunohistochemistry assay using the PD-L1 IHC 22C3 pharmDx kit and who had not received prior systemic treatment for metastatic NSCLC were eligible. Patients with EGFR or ALK genomic tumor aberrations; autoimmune disease that required systemic therapy within 2 years of treatment; a medical condition that required immunosuppression; or who had received more than 30 Gy of radiation in the thoracic region within the prior 26 weeks of initiation of study were ineligible. Randomization was stratified by ECOG PS (0 vs. 1), histology (squamous vs. non-squamous), geographic region (East Asia vs. non-East Asia), and PD-L1 expression (TPS ≥50% vs. TPS 1 to 49%). Patients were randomized (1:1) to receive KEYTRUDA 200 mg intravenously every 3 weeks or investigator's choice of either of the following platinum-containing chemotherapy regimens:

• Pemetrexed 500 mg/m2 every 3 weeks and carboplatin AUC 5 to 6 mg/mL/min every 3 weeks on Day 1 for a maximum of 6 cycles followed by optional pemetrexed 500 mg/m2 every 3 weeks for patients with nonsquamous histologies;

• Paclitaxel 200 mg/m2 every 3 weeks and carboplatin AUC 5 to 6 mg/mL/min every 3 weeks on Day 1 for a maximum of 6 cycles followed by optional pemetrexed 500 mg/m2 every 3 weeks for patients with non-squamous histologies. Treatment with KEYTRUDA continued until RECIST v1.1 (modified to follow a maximum of 10 target lesions and a maximum of 5 target lesions per organ)-defined progression of disease, unacceptable toxicity, or a maximum of 24 months. Administration of KEYTRUDA was permitted beyond RECIST defined disease progression if the patient was clinically stable and deriving clinical benefit as determined by the investigator. Treatment with KEYTRUDA could be reinitiated at the time of subsequent disease progression and administered for up to 12 months. Assessment of tumor status was performed every 9 weeks. The main efficacy outcome measure was OS in the subgroup of patients with TPS ≥50% NSCLC, the subgroup of patients with TPS ≥20% NSCLC, and the overall population with TPS ≥1% NSCLC. Additional efficacy outcome measures were PFS and ORR in the subgroup of patients with TPS ≥50% NSCLC, the subgroup of patients with TPS ≥20% NSCLC, and the overall population with TPS ≥1% NSCLC as assessed by BICR according to RECIST v1.1, modified to follow a maximum of 10 target lesions and a maximum of 5 target lesions per organ. The study population characteristics were: median age of 63 years (range: 25 to 90), 45% age 65 or older; 71% male; and 64% White, 30% Asian, and 2% Black. Nineteen percent were Hispanic or Latino. Sixty-nine percent had ECOG PS of 1; 39% with squamous and 61% with non-squamous histology; 87% had M1 disease and 13% had Stage IIIA (2%) or Stage IIIB (11%) and who were not candidates for surgical resection or definitive chemoradiation per investigator assessment; and 5% with treated brain metastases at baseline. Forty-seven percent of patients had TPS ≥50% NSCLC and 53% had TPS 1 to 49% NSCLC.

The trial demonstrated a statistically significant improvement in OS for patients (PD-L1 TPS ≥50%, TPS ≥20%, TPS ≥1%) randomized to KEYTRUDA as compared with chemotherapy.

The efficacy of KEYTRUDA was also investigated in KEYNOTE-024 (NCT02142738).

A randomized, multicenter, open-label, active-controlled trial in 305 previously untreated patients with metastatic NSCLC.

The study design was similar to that of KEYNOTE-042, except that only patients whose tumors had high PD-L1 expression (TPS of 50% or greater) by an immunohistochemistry assay using the PD-L1 IHC 22C3 pharmDx kit were eligible. Patients were randomized (1:1) to receive KEYTRUDA 200 mg intravenously every 3 weeks or investigator's choice of any of the following platinum-containing chemotherapy regimens:

• Pemetrexed 500 mg/m2 every 3 weeks and carboplatin AUC 5 to 6 mg/mL/min every 3 weeks on Day 1 for 4 to 6 cycles followed by optional pemetrexed 500 mg/m2 every 3 weeks for patients with nonsquamous histologies; • Pemetrexed 500 mg/m2 every 3 weeks and cisplatin 75 mg/m2 every 3 weeks on Day 1 for 4 to 6 cycles followed by optional pemetrexed 500 mg/m2 every 3 weeks for patients with non-squamous histologies;

• Gemcitabine 1250 mg/m2 on days 1 and 8 and cisplatin 75 mg/m2 every 3 weeks on Day 1 for 4 to 6 cycles;

• Gemcitabine 1250 mg/m2 on Days 1 and 8 and carboplatin AUC 5 to 6 mg/mL/min every 3 weeks on Day 1 for 4 to 6 cycles;

• Paclitaxel 200 mg/m2 every 3 weeks and carboplatin AUC 5 to 6 mg/mL/min every 3 weeks on Day 1 for 4 to 6 cycles followed by optional pemetrexed maintenance (for non-squamous histologies). Patients randomized to chemotherapy were offered KEYTRUDA at the time of disease progression.

The main efficacy outcome measure was PFS as assessed by BICR according to RECIST v1.1, modified to follow a maximum of 10 target lesions and a maximum of 5 target lesions per organ. Additional efficacy outcome measures were OS and ORR as assessed by BICR according to RECIST v1.1, modified to follow a maximum of 10 target lesions and a maximum of 5 target lesions per organ. The study population characteristics were: median age of 65 years (range: 33 to 90), 54% age 65 or older; 61% male; 82% White and 15% Asian; 65% with ECOG PS of 1; 18% with squamous and 82% with non-squamous histology and 9% with history of brain metastases. A total of 66 patients in the chemotherapy arm received KEYTRUDA at the time of disease progression.

The trial demonstrated a statistically significant improvement in both PFS and OS for patients randomized to KEYTRUDA as compared with chemotherapy.

Previously treated NSCLC

The efficacy of KEYTRUDA was investigated in KEYNOTE-010 (NCT01905657), a randomized, multicenter, open-label, active-controlled trial conducted in 1033 patients with metastatic NSCLC that had progressed following platinum-containing chemotherapy, and if appropriate, targeted therapy for EGFR or ALK genomic tumor aberrations. Eligible patients had PD-L1 expression TPS of 1% or greater by an immunohistochemistry assay using the PD-L1 IHC 22C3 pharmDx kit. Patients with autoimmune disease; a medical condition that required immunosuppression; or who had received more than 30 Gy of thoracic radiation within the prior 26 weeks were ineligible. Randomization was stratified by tumor PD-L1 expression (PD-L1 expression TPS ≥50% vs. PD-L1 expression TPS=1-49%), ECOG PS (0 vs. 1), and geographic region (East Asia vs. non-East Asia). Patients were randomized (1:1:1) to receive KEYTRUDA 2 mg/kg intravenously every 3 weeks, KEYTRUDA 10 mg/kg intravenously every 3 weeks or docetaxel intravenously 75 mg/m2 every 3 weeks until unacceptable toxicity or disease progression. Patients randomized to KEYTRUDA were permitted to continue until disease progression that was symptomatic, rapidly progressive, required urgent intervention, occurred with a decline in performance status, or confirmation of progression at 4 to 6 weeks with repeat imaging or for up to 24 months without disease progression. Assessment of tumor status was performed every 9 weeks. The main efficacy outcome measures were OS and PFS as assessed by BICR according to RECIST v1.1, modified to follow a maximum of 10 target lesions and a maximum of 5 target lesions per organ, in the subgroup of patients with TPS ≥50% and the overall population with TPS ≥1%. Additional efficacy outcome measures were ORR and DoR in the subgroup of patients with TPS ≥50% and the overall population with TPS ≥1%. The study population characteristics were: median age of 63 years (range: 20 to 88), 42% age 65 or older; 61% male; 72% White and 21% Asian; 66% ECOG PS of 1; 43% with high PD-L1 tumor expression; 21% with squamous, 70% with non-squamous, and 8% with mixed, other or unknown histology; 91% metastatic (M1) disease; 15% with history of brain metastases; and 8% and 1% with EGFR and ALK genomic aberrations, respectively. All patients had received prior therapy with a platinum doublet regimen, 29% received two or more prior therapies for their metastatic disease.

Neoadjuvant and adjuvant treatment of resectable NSCLC

The efficacy of KEYTRUDA in combination with neoadjuvant chemotherapy followed by surgery and continued adjuvant treatment with KEYTRUDA as a single agent was investigated in KEYNOTE-671 (NCT03425643), a multicenter, randomized, double-blind, placebo-controlled trial conducted in 797 patients with previously untreated and resectable Stage II, IIIA, or IIIB (N2) NSCLC by AJCC 8th edition. Patients were enrolled regardless of tumor PD-L1 expression. Patients with active autoimmune disease that required systemic therapy within 2 years of treatment, a medical condition that required immunosuppression, or a history of interstitial lung disease or pneumonitis that required steroids were ineligible. Randomization was stratified by stage (II vs. III), tumor PD-L1 expression (TPS ≥50% or <50%), histology (squamous vs. nonsquamous), and geographic region (East Asia vs. non-East Asia). Patients were randomized (1:1) to one of the following treatment arms:

• Treatment Arm A: neoadjuvant KEYTRUDA 200 mg on Day 1 in combination with cisplatin 75 mg/m2 and either pemetrexed 500 mg/m2 on Day 1 or gemcitabine 1000 mg/m2 on Days 1 and 8 of each 21-day cycle for up to 4 cycles. Within 4-12 weeks following surgery, KEYTRUDA 200 mg was administered every 3 weeks for up to 13 cycles.

• Treatment Arm B: neoadjuvant placebo on Day 1 in combination with cisplatin 75 mg/m2 and either pemetrexed 500 mg/m2 on Day 1 or gemcitabine 1000 mg/m2 on Days 1 and 8 of each 21-day cycle for up to 4 cycles. Within 4-12 weeks following surgery, placebo was administered every 3 weeks for up to 13 cycles. All study medications were administered via intravenous infusion. Treatment with KEYTRUDA or placebo continued until completion of the treatment (17 cycles), disease progression that precluded definitive surgery, disease recurrence in the adjuvant phase, disease progression for those who did not undergo surgery or had incomplete resection and entered the adjuvant phase, or unacceptable toxicity. Assessment of tumor status was performed at baseline, Week 7, and Week 13 in the neoadjuvant phase and within 4 weeks prior to the start of the adjuvant phase. Following the start of the adjuvant phase, assessment of tumor status was performed every 16 weeks through the end of Year 3, and then every 6 months thereafter. The trial was not designed to isolate the effect of KEYTRUDA in each phase (neoadjuvant or adjuvant) of treatment.

The major efficacy outcome measures were OS and investigator-assessed event-free survival (EFS). Additional efficacy outcome measures were pathological complete response (pCR) rate and major pathological response (mPR) rate as assessed by blinded independent pathology review.

The study population characteristics were: median age of 64 years (range: 26 to 83); 45% age 65 or older and 7% age 75 or older; 71% male; 61% White, 31% Asian, 2% Black, 4% race not reported; 9% Hispanic or Latino; 63% ECOG PS of 0 and 37% ECOG PS of 1. Thirty percent had Stage II and 70% had Stage III disease; 33% had TPS ≥50% and 67% had TPS <50%; 43% had tumors with squamous histology and 57% had tumors with non-squamous histology; 31% were from the East Asian region.

Eighty-one percent of patients in the KEYTRUDA in combination with platinum-containing chemotherapy arm received definitive surgery compared to 76% of patients in the placebo in combination with platinum-containing chemotherapy arm.

The trial demonstrated statistically significant improvements in OS and EFS for patients randomized to KEYTRUDA in combination with platinum-containing chemotherapy followed by KEYTRUDA as a single agent compared with patients randomized to placebo in combination with platinum-containing chemotherapy followed by placebo alone.

Adjuvant treatment of resected NSCLC

The efficacy of KEYTRUDA was investigated in KEYNOTE-091 (NCT02504372), a multicenter, randomized, triple-blind, placebo-controlled trial conducted in 1177 patients with completely resected Stage IB (T2a ≥4 cm), II, or IIIA NSCLC by AJCC 7th edition. Patients had not received neoadjuvant radiotherapy or chemotherapy.

Adjuvant chemotherapy up to 4 cycles was optional. Patients were ineligible if they had active autoimmune disease, were on chronic immunosuppressive agents, or had a history of interstitial lung disease or pneumonitis. Randomization was stratified by stage (IB vs. II vs. IIIA), receipt of adjuvant chemotherapy (yes vs. no), PD-L1 status (TPS <1% [negative] vs. TPS 1-49% vs. TPS ≥50%), and geographic region (Western Europe vs. Eastern Europe vs. Asia vs. Rest of World). Patients were randomized (1:1) to receive KEYTRUDA 200 mg or placebo intravenously every 3 weeks. Treatment continued until RECIST v1.1-defined disease recurrence as determined by the investigator, unacceptable toxicity or up to one year. Tumor assessments were conducted every 12 weeks for the first year, then every 6 months for years 2 to 3, and then annually through year 5. After year 5, imaging was 95 Reference ID: 5448057 performed as per local standard of care. The major efficacy outcome measure was investigator-assessed disease-free survival (DFS). An additional efficacy outcome measure was OS. Of 1177 patients randomized, 1010 (86%) received adjuvant platinum-based chemotherapy following resection. Among these 1010 patients, the median age was 64 years (range: 35 to 84), 49% age 65 or older; 68% male; 77% White, 18% Asian; 86% current or former smokers; and 39% with ECOG PS of 1. Eleven percent had Stage IB, 57% had Stage II, and 31% had Stage IIIA disease. Thirty-nine percent had PD-L1 TPS <1% [negative], 33% had TPS 1-49%, and 28% had TPS ≥50%. Fifty-two percent were from Western Europe, 20% from Eastern Europe, 17% from Asia, and 11% from Rest of World.

The trial met its primary endpoint, demonstrating a statistically significant improvement in DFS in the overall population for patients randomized to the KEYTRUDA arm compared to patients randomized to the placebo arm. In an exploratory subgroup analysis of the 167 patients (14%) who did not receive adjuvant chemotherapy, the DFS HR was 1.25 (95% CI: 0.76, 2.05). OS results were not mature with only 42% of pre-specified OS events in the overall population.

14.3 Malignant Pleural Mesothelioma

First-line treatment of unresectable advanced or metastatic malignant pleural mesothelioma (MPM) with pemetrexed and platinum chemotherapy.

The efficacy of KEYTRUDA in combination with pemetrexed and platinum chemotherapy was investigated in KEYNOTE-483 (NCT02784171), a multicenter, randomized, open-label, active-controlled trial that enrolled 440 patients with unresectable advanced or metastatic MPM and no prior systemic therapy for advanced/metastatic disease. Patients were enrolled regardless of tumor PD-L1 expression. Patients with autoimmune disease that required systemic therapy within 3 years of treatment or a medical condition that required immunosuppression were ineligible. Randomization was stratified by histological subtype (epithelioid vs. non-epithelioid). Patients were randomized (1:1) to one of the following treatment arms; all study medications were administered via intravenous infusion:

- KEYTRUDA 200 mg with pemetrexed 500 mg/m2 and cisplatin 75 mg/m2 or carboplatin AUC 5-6 mg/mL/min on Day 1 of each 21-day cycle for up to 6 cycles, followed by KEYTRUDA 200 mg every 3 weeks. KEYTRUDA was administered prior to chemotherapy on Day 1.

- Pemetrexed 500 mg/m2 and cisplatin 75 mg/m2 or carboplatin AUC 5-6 mg/mL/min on Day 1 of each 21-day cycle for up to 6 cycles. Treatment with KEYTRUDA continued until disease progression as determined by the investigator according to modified RECIST 1.1 for mesothelioma (mRECIST), unacceptable toxicity, or a maximum of 24 months. Assessment of tumor status was performed every 6 weeks for 18 weeks, followed by every 12 weeks thereafter. The main efficacy outcome measure was OS. Additional efficacy outcome measures were PFS, ORR, and DoR, as assessed by BICR according to mRECIST. The study population characteristics were: median age of 70 years (77% age 65 or older); 76% male; 79% White, 21% race not reported or unknown; 2% Hispanic or Latino; and 53% ECOG performance status of 1. Seventy-eight percent had epithelioid and 22% had non-epithelioid histology; 60% had tumors with PD-L1 CPS ≥1 and 30% had tumors with PD-L1 CPS equal to, or greater than, 1 and 30% had tumors with PD-L1 CPS <1.

The trial demonstrated a statistically significant improvement in OS, PFS, and ORR in patients randomized to KEYTRUDA in combination with chemotherapy compared with patients randomized to chemotherapy alone.

(*Figure 44. Diffuse pleural mesothelioma with extensive involvement of the pericardium)*

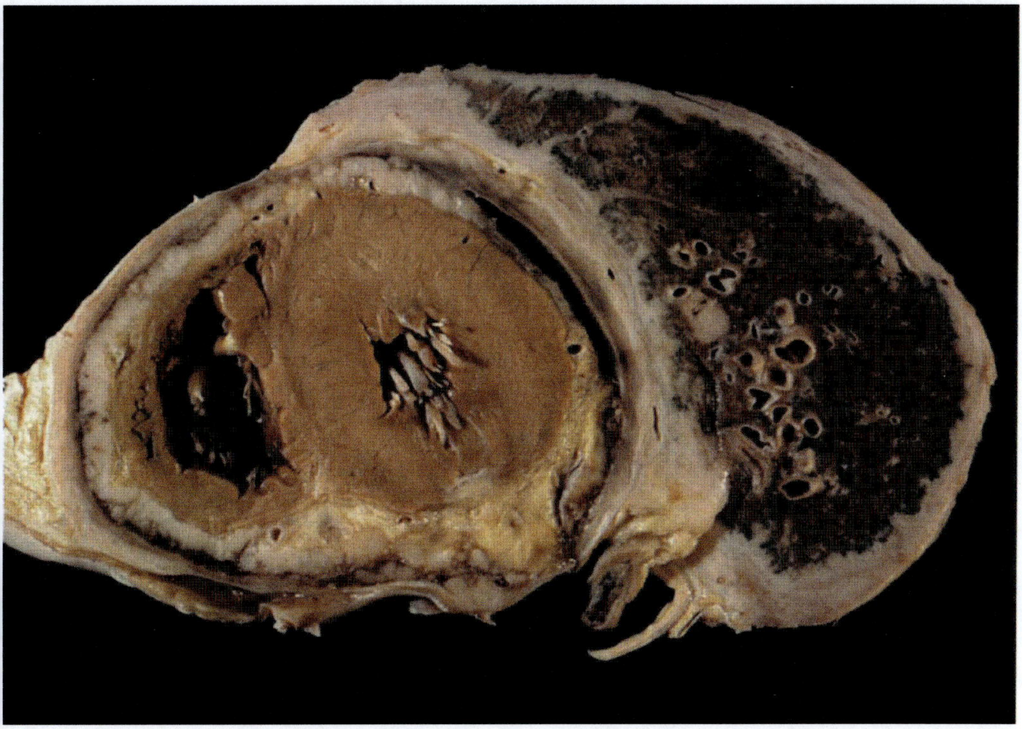

(This image is by The Armed Forces Institute of Pathology (AFIP) - PEIR Digital Library (Pathology image database). Image# 410524. Public Domain, https://commons.wikimedia.org/w/index.php?curid=4337356; https://en.wikipedia.org/wiki/Mesothelioma#/media/File:Diffuse_pleural_mesothelioma.jpg. This work is in the public domain in the United States because it is a work prepared by an officer or employee of the United States Government as part of that person's official duties under the terms of Title 17, Chapter 1, Section 105 of the US Code.. No changes were made to this image).

(Figure 45. Photomicrographs showing conventionally-stained mesothelioma in a core biopsy (higher magnifications on right).

This image is by Robertolyra - Own work, Public Domain, https://commons.wikimedia.org/w/index.php?curid=7093479; n.wikipedia.org/wiki/Mesothelioma#/media/File:Mesothelioma.PNG. The copyright holder of this work, release this work into the public domain. No changes were made to this image).

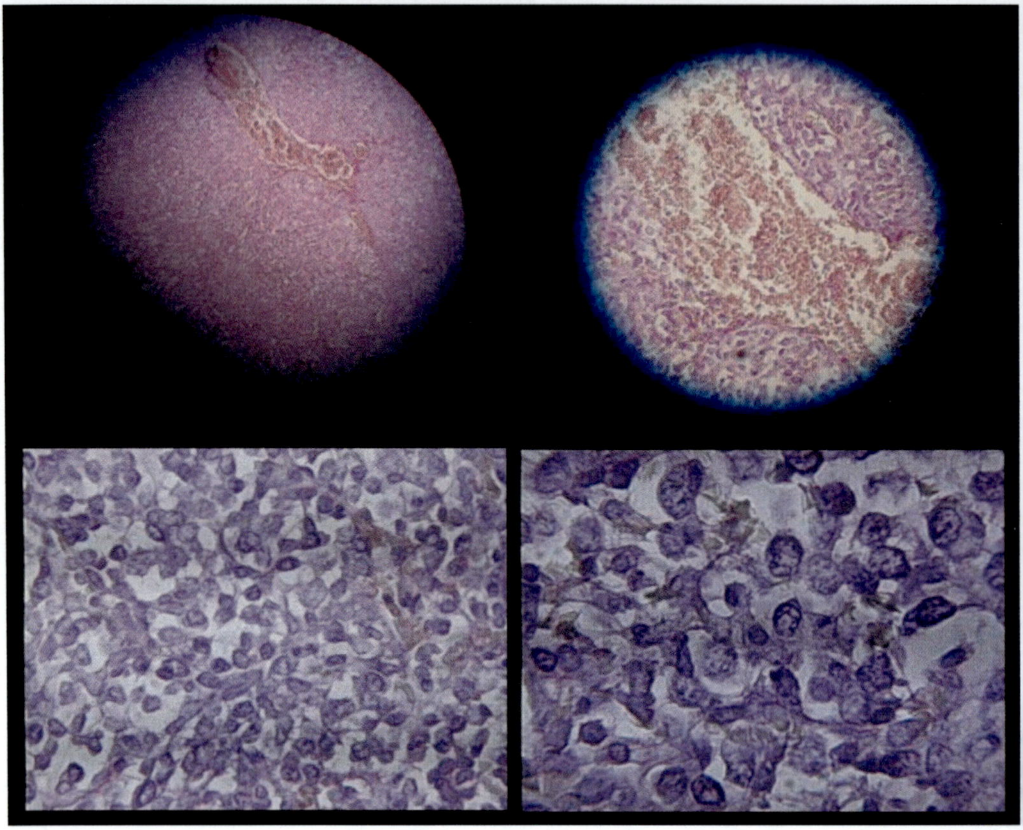

14.4 Head and Neck Squamous Cell Cancer (HNSCC)

First-line treatment of metastatic or unresectable, recurrent HNSCC

The efficacy of KEYTRUDA was investigated in KEYNOTE-048 (NCT02358031), a randomized, multicenter, open-label, active-controlled trial conducted in 882 patients with metastatic HNSCC who had not previously received systemic therapy for metastatic disease or with recurrent disease who were considered incurable by local therapies. Patients with active autoimmune disease that required systemic therapy within two years of treatment or a medical condition that required immunosuppression were ineligible. Randomization was stratified by tumor PD-L1 expression (TPS ≥50% or <50%) according to the PD-L1 IHC 22C3 pharmDx kit, HPV status according to p16 IHC (positive or negative), and ECOG PS (0 vs. 1). Patients were randomized 1:1:1 to one of the following treatment arms:

• KEYTRUDA 200 mg intravenously every 3 weeks

• KEYTRUDA 200 mg intravenously every 3 weeks, carboplatin AUC 5 mg/mL/min intravenously every 3 weeks or cisplatin 100 mg/m2 intravenously every 3 weeks, and FU 1000 mg/m2/day as a continuous intravenous infusion over 96 hours every 3 weeks (maximum of 6 cycles of platinum and FU)

• Cetuximab 400 mg/m2 intravenously as the initial dose then 250 mg/m2 intravenously once weekly, carboplatin AUC 5 mg/mL/min intravenously every 3 weeks or cisplatin 100 mg/m2 intravenously every 3 weeks, and FU 1000 mg/m2/day as a continuous intravenous infusion over 96 hours every 3 weeks (maximum of 6 cycles of platinum and FU). Treatment with KEYTRUDA continued until RECIST v1.1-defined progression of disease as determined by the investigator, unacceptable toxicity, or a maximum of 24 months. Administration of KEYTRUDA was permitted beyond RECIST-defined disease progression if the patient was clinically stable and considered to be deriving clinical benefit by the investigator. Assessment of tumor status was performed at Week 9 and then every 6 weeks for the first year, followed by every 9 weeks through 24 months. A retrospective re-classification of patients' tumor PD-L1 status according to CPS using the PD-L1 IHC 22C3 pharmDx kit was conducted using the tumor specimens used for randomization. The main efficacy outcome measures were OS and PFS as assessed by BICR according to RECIST v1.1 (modified to follow a maximum of 10 target lesions and a maximum of 5 target lesions per organ) sequentially tested in the subgroup of patients with CPS ≥20, the subgroup of patients with CPS ≥1, and the overall population.

The study population characteristics were: median age of 61 years (range: 20 to 94), 36% age 65 or older; 83% male; 73% White, 20% Asian and 2.4% Black; 61% had ECOG PS of 1; and 79% were former/current smokers. Twenty-two percent of patients' tumors were HPV-positive, 23% had PD-L1 TPS ≥50%, and 95% had Stage IV disease (Stage IVA 19%, Stage IVB 6%, and Stage IVC 70%). Eighty-five percent of patients' tumors had PD-L1 expression of CPS ≥1 and 43% had CPS ≥20.

The trial demonstrated a statistically significant improvement in OS for patients randomized to KEYTRUDA in combination with chemotherapy compared to those randomized to cetuximab in combination with chemotherapy at a pre-specified interim analysis in the overall population.

Previously treated recurrent or metastatic HNSCC

The efficacy of KEYTRUDA was investigated in KEYNOTE-012 (NCT01848834), a multicenter, non randomized, open-label, multi-cohort study that enrolled 174 patients with recurrent or metastatic HNSCC who had disease progression on or after platinum-containing chemotherapy administered for recurrent or metastatic HNSCC or following platinum-containing chemotherapy administered as part of induction, concurrent, or adjuvant therapy. Patients with active autoimmune disease, a medical condition that required immunosuppression, evidence of interstitial lung disease, or ECOG PS ≥2 were ineligible.

Patients received KEYTRUDA 10 mg/kg every 2 weeks (n=53) or 200 mg every 3 weeks (n=121) until unacceptable toxicity or disease progression that was symptomatic, was rapidly progressive, required urgent intervention, occurred with a decline in performance status, or was confirmed at least 4 weeks later with repeat imaging. Patients without disease progression were treated for up to 24 months. Treatment with pembrolizumab could be reinitiated for subsequent disease progression and administered for up to 1 additional year.

Assessment of tumor status was performed every 8 weeks. The major efficacy outcome measures were ORR according to RECIST v1.1, modified to follow a maximum of 10 target lesions and a maximum of 5 target lesions per organ, as assessed by BICR, and DoR. The study population characteristics were median age of 60 years, 32% age 65 or older; 82% male; 75% White, 16% Asian, and 6% Black; 87% had M1 disease; 33% had HPV positive tumors; 63% had prior cetuximab; 29% had an ECOG PS of 0 and 71% had an ECOG PS of 1; and the median number of prior lines of therapy administered for the treatment of HNSCC was 2.

The ORR was 16% (95% CI: 11, 22) with a complete response rate of 5%. The median follow-up time was 8.9 months. Among the 28 responding patients, the median DoR had not been reached (range: 2.4+ to 27.7+ months), with 23 patients having responses of 6 months or longer. The ORR and DoR were similar irrespective of dosage regimen (10 mg/kg every 2 weeks or 200 mg every 3 weeks) or HPV status.

14.5 Classical Hodgkin Lymphoma (cHL)

The efficacy of KEYTRUDA was investigated in KEYNOTE-204 (NCT02684292), a randomized, open label, active controlled trial conducted in 304 patients with relapsed or refractory cHL. The trial enrolled adults with relapsed or refractory disease after at least one multi-agent chemotherapy regimen. Patients were randomized (1:1) to receive:

- KEYTRUDA 200 mg intravenously every 3 weeks or
- Brentuximab vedotin (BV) 1.8 mg/kg intravenously every 3 weeks

Treatment was continued until unacceptable toxicity, disease progression, or a maximum of 35 cycles (up to approximately 2 years). Disease assessment was performed every 12 weeks. Randomization was stratified by prior autologous HSCT (yes vs. no) and disease status after frontline therapy (primary refractory vs. relapse < 12 months after completion vs. relapse ≥12 months after completion).

The main efficacy measure was PFS as assessed by BICR using 2007 revised International Working Group criteria. The study population characteristics were: median age of 35 years (range: 18 to 84); 57% male; 77% White, 9% Asian, 3.9% Black. The median number of prior therapies was 2 (range: 1 to 10) in the KEYTRUDA arm and 3 (range: 1 to 11) in the BV arm, with 18% in both arms having 1 prior line. Forty two percent of patients were refractory to the last prior therapy, 29% had primary refractory disease, 37% had prior autologous HSCT, 5% had received prior BV, and 39% had prior radiation therapy.

The objective response rate significantly favored KEYTRUDA.

KEYNOTE-087 (NCT02453594), a multicenter, non randomized, open-label trial in 210 patients with relapsed or refractory cHL.

The efficacy of KEYTRUDA was investigated in KEYNOTE-087 (NCT02453594), a multicenter, non randomized, open-label trial in 210 patients with relapsed or refractory cHL. Patients with active, non-infectious pneumonitis, an allogeneic HSCT within the past 5 years (or >5 years but with symptoms of GVHD), active autoimmune disease, a medical condition that required immunosuppression, or an active infection requiring systemic therapy were ineligible for the trial.

Patients received KEYTRUDA 200 mg intravenously every 3 weeks until unacceptable toxicity or documented disease progression, or for up to 24 months in patients who did not progress. Disease assessment was performed every 12 weeks. The major efficacy outcome measures (ORR, Complete Response Rate, and DoR) were assessed by BICR according to the 2007 revised International Working Group (IWG) criteria.

The study population characteristics were: median age of 35 years (range: 18 to 76), 9% age 65 or older; 54% male; 88% White; and 49% ECOG PS of 0 and 51% ECOG PS of 1. The median number of prior lines of therapy administered for the treatment of cHL was 4 (range: 1 to 12). Fifty-eight percent were refractory to the last prior therapy, including 35% with primary refractory disease and 14% whose disease was chemo-refractory to all prior regimens. Sixty-one percent of patients had undergone prior autologous HSCT, 83% had received prior brentuximab vedotin and 36% of patients had prior radiation therapy.

The objective response rate was 69% and the median duration of response was 11.1 months.

14.6 Primary Mediastinal Large B-Cell Lymphoma (PMBCL)

The efficacy of KEYTRUDA was investigated in KEYNOTE-170 (NCT02576990), a multicenter, open label, single-arm trial in 53 patients with relapsed or refractory PMBCL. Patients were not eligible if they had active non-infectious pneumonitis, allogeneic HSCT within the past 5 years (or >5 years but with symptoms of GVHD), active autoimmune disease, a medical condition that required immunosuppression, or an active infection requiring systemic therapy.

Patients were treated with KEYTRUDA 200 mg intravenously every 3 weeks until unacceptable toxicity or documented disease progression, or for up to 24 months for patients who did not progress. Disease assessments were performed every 12 weeks and assessed by BICR according to the 2007 revised IWG criteria. The efficacy outcome measures were ORR and DoR.

The study population characteristics were: median age of 33 years (range: 20 to 61 years); 43% male; 92% White; and 43% ECOG PS of 0 and 57% ECOG PS of 1. The median number of prior lines of therapy administered for the treatment of

PMBCL was 3 (range 2 to 8). Thirty-six percent had primary refractory disease, 49% had relapsed disease refractory to the last prior therapy, and 15% had untreated relapse. Twenty-six percent of patients had undergone prior autologous HSCT, and 32% of patients had prior radiation therapy. All patients had received rituximab as part of a prior line of therapy. For the 24 responders, the median time to first objective response (complete or partial response) was 2.8 months (range 2.1 to 8.5 months).

The objective response rate was 45% and the median duration of response was not reached (range: 1.1+ to 19.2+ months).

14.7 Urothelial Cancer

In Combination with Enfortumab Vedotin for the Treatment of Patients with Urothelial Cancer

The efficacy of KEYTRUDA in combination with enfortumab vedotin was evaluated in KEYNOTE-A39 (NCT04223856), an open-label, randomized, multicenter trial that enrolled 886 patients with locally advanced or metastatic urothelial cancer who received no prior systemic therapy for locally advanced or metastatic disease. Patients with active CNS metastases, ongoing sensory or motor neuropathy Grade ≥2, or uncontrolled diabetes defined as hemoglobin A1C (HbA1c) ≥8% or HbA1c ≥7% with associated diabetes symptoms were excluded. Patients were randomized 1:1 to receive either:

KEYTRUDA 200 mg over 30 minutes on Day 1 and enfortumab vedotin 1.25 mg/kg on Days 1 and 8 of each 21-day cycle.

KEYTRUDA was given approximately 30 minutes after enfortumab vedotin. Treatment was continued until disease progression or unacceptable toxicity. In the absence of disease progression or unacceptable toxicity, KEYTRUDA was continued for up to 2 years.

• Gemcitabine 1000 mg/m2 on Days 1 and 8 of a 21-day cycle with cisplatin 70 mg/m2 or carboplatin (AUC = 4.5 or 5) on Day 1 of a 21-day cycle. Treatment was continued until disease progression or unacceptable toxicity for up to 6 cycles. Randomization was stratified by cisplatin eligibility, PD-L1 expression, and presence of liver metastases. The median age was 69 years (range: 22 to 91); 77% were male; 67% were White, 22% were Asian, 1% were Black or African American, and 10% were unknown or other; 12% were Hispanic or Latino. Patients had a baseline ECOG performance status of 0 (49%), 1 (47%), or 2 (3%). Forty-seven percent of patients had a documented baseline HbA1c of <5.7%. At baseline, 95% of patients had metastatic urothelial cancer, including 72% with visceral and 22% with liver metastases, and 5% had locally advanced urothelial cancer. Eighty-five percent of patients had urothelial carcinoma (UC) histology including 6% with UC mixed squamous differentiation and 2% with UC mixed other histologic variants. Forty-six percent of patients were considered cisplatin-ineligible and 54% were considered cisplatin-eligible at time of randomization.

The major efficacy outcome measures were OS and PFS as assessed by BICR according to RECIST v1.1. Additional efficacy outcome measures included ORR as assessed by BICR. The trial demonstrated statistically significant improvements in OS, PFS, and ORR for patients randomized to KEYTRUDA in combination with enfortumab vedotin as compared to platinum-based chemotherapy. Efficacy results were consistent across all stratified patient subgroups.

In Combination with Enfortumab Vedotin for the Treatment of Cisplatin-Ineligible Patients with Urothelial Cancer

The efficacy of KEYTRUDA in combination with enfortumab vedotin was evaluated in KEYNOTE-869 (NCT03288545), an open-label, multi-cohort (dose escalation cohort, Cohort A, Cohort K) study in patients with locally advanced or metastatic urothelial cancer who were ineligible for cisplatin-containing chemotherapy and received no prior systemic therapy for locally advanced or metastatic disease. Patients with active CNS metastases, ongoing sensory or motor neuropathy Grade ≥2, or uncontrolled diabetes defined as hemoglobin A1C (HbA1c) ≥8% or HbA1c ≥7% with associated diabetes symptoms were excluded from participating in the study. Patients in the dose escalation cohort (n=5), Cohort A (n=40), and Cohort K (n=76) received enfortumab vedotin 1.25 mg/kg as an IV infusion over 30 minutes on Days 1 and 8 of a 21-day cycle followed by KEYTRUDA 200 mg as an IV infusion on Day 1 of a 21-day cycle approximately 30 minutes after enfortumab vedotin. Patients were treated until disease progression or unacceptable toxicity. A total of 121 patients received KEYTRUDA in combination with enfortumab vedotin. The median age was 71 years (range: 51 to 91); 74% were male; 85% were White, 5% were Black, 4% were Asian and 6% were other, unknown or not reported. Ten percent of patients were Hispanic or Latino. Forty-five percent of patients had an ECOG performance status of 1 and 15% had an ECOG performance status of 2. Forty-seven percent of patients had a documented baseline HbA1c of <5.7%. Reasons for cisplatin-ineligibility included: 60% with baseline creatinine clearance of 30-59 mL/min, 10% with ECOG PS of 2, 13% with Grade 2 or greater hearing loss, and 16% with more than one cisplatin-ineligibility criteria. At baseline, 97.5% of patients had metastatic urothelial cancer and 2.5% of patients had locally advanced urothelial cancer. Thirty-seven percent of patients had upper tract disease. Eighty-four percent of patients had visceral metastasis at baseline, including 22% with liver metastases. Thirty-nine percent of patients had TCC histology; 13% had TCC with squamous differentiation, and 48% had TCC with other histologic variants.

The major efficacy outcome measures were ORR and DoR as assessed by BICR according to RECIST v1.1. The median follow-up time for the dose escalation cohort + Cohort A was 44.7 months (range 0.7 to 52.4) and for Cohort K was 14.8 months.(range: 0.6 to 26.2).

The objective response rate was 68%.

Platinum-Ineligible Patients with Urothelial Carcinoma

The efficacy of KEYTRUDA was investigated in KEYNOTE-052 (NCT02335424), a multicenter, open label, single-arm trial in 370 patients with locally advanced or metastatic urothelial carcinoma who had one or more comorbidities, including patients who were not eligible for any platinum-containing chemotherapy. The trial excluded patients with autoimmune disease or a medical condition that required immunosuppression.

Patients received KEYTRUDA 200 mg every 3 weeks until unacceptable toxicity or disease progression. Patients with initial radiographic disease progression could receive additional doses of treatment during confirmation of progression unless disease progression was symptomatic, was rapidly progressive, required urgent intervention, or occurred with a decline in performance status. Patients without disease progression could be treated for up to 24 months.

Tumor response assessments were performed at 9 weeks after the first dose, then every 6 weeks for the first year, and then every 12 weeks thereafter. The major efficacy outcome measures were ORR and DoR as assessed by BICR according to RECIST v1.1, modified to follow a maximum of 10 target lesions and a maximum of 5 target lesions per organ. The study population characteristics were: median age of 74 years; 77% male; and 89% White. Eighty seven percent had M1 disease, and 13% had M0 disease. Eighty-one percent had a primary tumor in the lower tract, and 19% of patients had a primary tumor in the upper tract. Eighty-five percent of patients had visceral metastases, including 21% with liver metastases. Fifty percent of patients had baseline creatinine clearance of <60 mL/min, 32% had ECOG PS of 2, 9% had ECOG PS of 2 and baseline creatinine clearance of <60 mL/min, and 9% had one or more of Class III heart failure, Grade 2 or greater peripheral neuropathy, and Grade 2 or greater hearing loss. Ninety percent of patients were treatment naïve, and 10% received prior adjuvant or neoadjuvant platinum-based chemotherapy. The median follow-up time for 370 patients treated with KEYTRUDA was 11.4 months (range 0.1 to 63.8 months).

The objective response rate was 29% and the median duration of response was 33.4 months (range 1.4+ to 60.7+).

Platinum-Eligible Patients with Previously Untreated Urothelial Carcinoma

The efficacy of KEYTRUDA for the first-line treatment of platinum-eligible patients with locally advanced or metastatic urothelial carcinoma was investigated in KEYNOTE-361 (NCT02853305), a multicenter, randomized, open-label, active-controlled study in 1010 previously untreated patients. The safety and efficacy of KEYTRUDA in combination with platinum-based chemotherapy for previously untreated patients with locally advanced or metastatic urothelial carcinoma has not been established.

The study compared KEYTRUDA with or without platinum-based chemotherapy (i.e., cisplatin or carboplatin with gemcitabine) to platinum-based chemotherapy alone. Among the patients receiving KEYTRUDA plus platinum-based chemotherapy, 44% received cisplatin and 56% received carboplatin.

The study did not meet its major efficacy outcome measures of improved PFS or OS in the KEYTRUDA plus chemotherapy arm compared to the chemotherapy-alone arm. Additional efficacy endpoints, including improvement of OS in the KEYTRUDA monotherapy arm, could not be formally tested.

Previously Treated Urothelial Carcinoma

The efficacy of KEYTRUDA was investigated in KEYNOTE-045 (NCT02256436), a multicenter, randomized (1:1), active-controlled trial in 542 patients with locally advanced or metastatic urothelial carcinoma with disease progression on or after platinum-containing chemotherapy. The trial excluded patients with autoimmune disease or a medical condition that required immunosuppression.

Patients were randomized to receive either KEYTRUDA 200 mg every 3 weeks (n=270) or investigator's choice of any of the following chemotherapy regimens all given intravenously every 3 weeks (n=272): paclitaxel 175 mg/m^2 (n=90), docetaxel 75 mg/m^2 (n=92), or vinflunine 320 mg/m^2 (n=90). Treatment continued until unacceptable toxicity or disease progression. Patients with initial radiographic disease progression could receive additional doses of treatment during confirmation of progression unless disease progression was symptomatic, was rapidly progressive, required urgent intervention, or occurred with a decline in performance status. Patients without disease progression could be treated for up to 24 months. Assessment of tumor status was performed at 9 weeks after randomization, then every 6 weeks through the first year, followed by every 12 weeks thereafter.

The major efficacy outcomes were OS and PFS as assessed by BICR per RECIST v1.1, modified to follow a maximum of 10 target lesions and a maximum of 5 target lesions per organ. Additional efficacy outcome measures were ORR as assessed by BICR per RECIST v1.1, modified to follow a maximum of 10 target lesions and a maximum of 5 target lesions per organ, and DoR.

The study population characteristics were: median age of 66 years (range: 26 to 88), 58% age 65 or older; 74% male; 72% White and 23% Asian; 42% ECOG PS of 0 and 56% ECOG PS of 1; and 96% M1 disease and 4% M0 disease. Eighty-seven percent of patients had visceral metastases, including 34% with liver metastases. Eighty-six percent had a primary tumor in the lower tract and 14% had a primary tumor in the upper tract. Fifteen percent of patients had disease progression following prior platinum containing neoadjuvant or adjuvant chemotherapy. Twenty-one percent had received 2 or more prior systemic regimens in the metastatic setting. Seventy-six percent of patients received prior cisplatin, 23% had prior carboplatin, and 1% were treated with other platinum-based regimens.

The study demonstrated statistically significant improvements in OS and ORR for patients randomized to KEYTRUDA as compared to chemotherapy. There was no statistically significant difference between KEYTRUDA and chemotherapy with respect to PFS. The median follow-up time for this trial was 9.0 months (range: 0.2 to 20.8 months).

BCG-unresponsive High-Risk Non-Muscle Invasive Bladder Cancer

The efficacy of KEYTRUDA was investigated in KEYNOTE-057 (NCT02625961), a multicenter, open label, single-arm trial in 96 patients with Bacillus Calmette-Guerin (BCG)-unresponsive, high-risk, non-muscle invasive bladder cancer (NMIBC) with carcinoma in situ (CIS) with or without papillary tumors who are ineligible for or have elected not to undergo cystectomy. BCG-unresponsive high-risk NMIBC was defined as persistent disease despite adequate BCG therapy, disease recurrence after an initial tumor-free state following adequate BCG therapy, or T1 disease following a single induction course of BCG. Adequate BCG therapy was defined as administration of at least five of six doses of an initial induction course plus either of: at least two of three doses of maintenance therapy or at least two of six doses of a second induction course. Prior to treatment, all patients had undergone transurethral resection of bladder tumor (TURBT) to remove all resectable disease (Ta and T1 components). Residual CIS (Tis components) not amenable to complete resection was allowed. The trial excluded patients with muscle-invasive (i.e., T2, T3, T4) locally advanced non-resectable or metastatic urothelial carcinoma, concurrent extra-vesical (i.e., urethra, ureter or renal pelvis) non-muscle invasive transitional cell carcinoma of the urothelium, or autoimmune disease or a medical condition that required immunosuppression.

Patients received KEYTRUDA 200 mg every 3 weeks until unacceptable toxicity, persistent or recurrent high-risk NMIBC, or progressive disease. Assessment of tumor status was performed every 12 weeks for two years and then every 24 weeks for three years, and patients without disease progression could be treated for up to 24 months. The major efficacy outcome measures were complete response (as defined by negative results for cystoscopy [with TURBT/biopsies as applicable], urine cytology, and computed tomography urography [CTU] imaging) and duration of response.

The study population characteristics were: median age of 73 years (range: 44 to 92); 44% age ≥75; 84% male; 67% White; and 73% and 27% with an ECOG performance status of 0 or 1, respectively. Tumor pattern at study entry was CIS with T1 (13%), CIS with high grade TA (25%), and CIS (63%). Baseline high-risk NMIBC disease status was 27% persistent and 73% recurrent. The median number of prior instillations of BCG was 12. The median follow-up time was 28.0 months (range: 4.6 to 40.5 months).

The objective response rate was 41% and the median duration of response was 16.2 months (range 0.0+ to 30.4+).

14.8. Microsatellite Instability-High or Mismatch Repair Deficient Cancer

The efficacy of KEYTRUDA was investigated in 504 patients with MSI-H or dMMR cancers enrolled in three multicenter, non-randomized, open-label, multi-cohort trials: KEYNOTE-164 (NCT02460198), KEYNOTE-158 (NCT02628067), and KEYNOTE-051 (NCT02332668). All trials excluded patients with autoimmune disease or a medical condition that required immunosuppression. Regardless of histology, MSI or MMR tumor status was determined using polymerase chain reaction (PCR; local or central) or immunohistochemistry (IHC; local or central), respectively.

- KEYNOTE-164 enrolled 124 patients with advanced MSI-H or dMMR colorectal cancer (CRC) that progressed following treatment with fluoropyrimidine and either oxaliplatin or irinotecan +/- anti-VEGF/EGFR mAb-based therapy.

- KEYNOTE-158 enrolled 373 patients with advanced MSI-H or dMMR non-colorectal cancers (non-CRC) who had disease progression following prior therapy. Patients were either prospectively enrolled with MSI-H/dMMR tumors (Cohort K) or retrospectively identified in one of 10 solid tumor cohorts (Cohorts A-J).

- KEYNOTE-051 enrolled 7 pediatric patients with MSI-H or dMMR cancers.

Adult patients received KEYTRUDA 200 mg every 3 weeks (pediatric patients received 2 mg/kg every 3 weeks) until unacceptable toxicity, disease progression, or a maximum of 24 months. In KEYNOTE-164 and KEYNOTE-158, assessment of tumor status was performed every 9 weeks through the first year, then every 12 weeks thereafter. In KEYNOTE-051, assessment of tumor status was performed every 8 weeks for 24 weeks, and then every 12 weeks thereafter.

The major efficacy outcome measures were ORR and DoR as assessed by BICR according to RECIST v1.1 (modified to follow a maximum of 10 target lesions and a maximum of 5 target lesions per organ in KEYNOTE-158) and as assessed by the investigator according to RECIST v1.1 in KEYNOTE-051.

In KEYNOTE-164 and KEYNOTE-158, the study population characteristics were median age of 60 years, 36% age 65 or older; 44% male; 78% White, 14% Asian, 4% American Indian or Alaska Native, and 3% Black; and 45% ECOG PS of 0 and 55% ECOG PS of 1. Ninety-two percent of patients had metastatic disease and 4% had locally advanced, unresectable disease. Thirty-seven percent of patients received one prior line of therapy and 61% received two or more prior lines of therapy.

In KEYNOTE-051, the study population characteristics were median age of 11 years (range: 3 to 16); 71% female; 86% White and 14% Asian; and 57% had a Lansky/Karnofsky Score of 100. Seventy-one percent of patients had Stage IV and 14% had Stage III disease. Fifty-seven percent of patients received one prior line of therapy and 29% received two prior lines of therapy. Discordant results were observed between local MSI-H or dMMR tests and central testing among patients enrolled in Cohort K of KEYNOTE-158. Among 104 tumor samples that were MSI-H or dMMR by local testing and also tested using the FoundationOne®CDx (F1CDx) test, 59 (56.7%) were MSI-H and 45 (43.3%) were not MSI-H. Among 169 tumor samples that were MSI-H or dMMR by local testing and also tested using the VENTANA MMR RxDx Panel, 105 (62.1%) were dMMR and 64 (37.9%) were pMMR.

The objective response rate was 33.3% and the median duration of response was 63.2 months (range 1.9+ to 63.9+).

14.9. Microsatellite Instability-High or Mismatch Repair Deficient Cancer

The efficacy of KEYTRUDA was investigated in KEYNOTE-177 (NCT02563002), a multicenter, randomized, open-label, active-controlled trial that enrolled 307 patients with previously untreated unresectable or metastatic MSI-H or dMMR CRC. MSI or

MMR tumor status was determined locally using polymerase chain reaction (PCR) or immunohistochemistry (IHC), respectively. Patients with autoimmune disease or a medical condition that required immunosuppression were ineligible. Patients were randomized (1:1) to receive KEYTRUDA 200 mg intravenously every 3 weeks or investigator's choice of the following chemotherapy regimens given intravenously every 2 weeks:

- mFOLFOX6 (oxaliplatin, leucovorin, and FU) or mFOLFOX6 in combination with either bevacizumab or cetuximab: Oxaliplatin 85 mg/m^2, leucovorin 400 mg/m^2 (or levoleucovorin 200 mg/m^2), and FU 400 mg/m^2 bolus on Day 1, then FU 2400 mg/m^2 over 46-48 hours. Bevacizumab 5 mg/kg on Day 1 or cetuximab 400 mg/m^2 on first infusion, then 250 mg/m2 weekly.

- FOLFIRI (irinotecan, leucovorin, and FU) or FOLFIRI in combination with either bevacizumab or cetuximab: Irinotecan 180 mg/m^2, leucovorin 400 mg/m^2 (or levoleucovorin 200 mg/m^2), and FU 400 mg/m^2 bolus on Day 1, then FU 2400 mg/m^2 over 46-48 hours. Bevacizumab 5 mg/kg on Day 1 or cetuximab 400 mg/m^2 on first infusion, then 250 mg/m^2 weekly.

Treatment with KEYTRUDA or chemotherapy continued until RECIST v1.1-defined progression of disease as determined by the investigator or unacceptable toxicity. Patients treated with KEYTRUDA without disease progression could be treated for up to 24 months. Assessment of tumor status was performed every 9 weeks. Patients randomized to chemotherapy were offered KEYTRUDA at the time of disease progression.

The main efficacy outcome measures were PFS (as assessed by BICR according to RECIST v1.1, modified to follow a maximum of 10 target lesions and a maximum of 5 target lesions per organ) and OS. Additional efficacy outcome measures were ORR and DoR. A total of 307 patients were enrolled and randomized to KEYTRUDA (n=153) or chemotherapy (n=154). The baseline characteristics of these 307 patients were: median age of 63 years (range: 24 to 93), 47% age 65 or older; 50% male; 75% White and 16% Asian; 52% had an ECOG PS of 0 and 48% had an ECOG PS of 1; and 27% received prior adjuvant or neoadjuvant chemotherapy. Among 154 patients randomized to receive chemotherapy,143 received chemotherapy per the protocol. Of the 143 patients, 56% received mFOLFOX6, 44% received FOLFIRI,

70% received bevacizumab plus mFOLFOX6 or FOLFIRI, and 11% received cetuximab plus mFOLFOX6 or FOLFIRI.

The trial demonstrated a statistically significant improvement in PFS for patients randomized to KEYTRUDA compared with chemotherapy. There was no statistically significant difference between KEYTRUDA and chemotherapy in the final OS analysis. Sixty percent of the patients who had been randomized to receive chemotherapy had crossed over to receive subsequent anti-PD-1/PD-L1 therapies including KEYTRUDA. The median follow-up time at the final analysis was 38.1 months (range: 0.2 to 58.7 months).

14.10. Gastric Cancer

First-line Treatment of Locally Advanced Unresectable or Metastatic HER2-Positive Gastric or Gastroesophageal Junction Adenocarcinoma

The efficacy of KEYTRUDA in combination with trastuzumab plus fluoropyrimidine and platinum chemotherapy was investigated in KEYNOTE-811 (NCT03615326), a multicenter, randomized, double-blind, placebo-controlled trial that enrolled 698 patients with HER2-positive advanced gastric or gastroesophageal junction (GEJ) adenocarcinoma who had not previously received systemic therapy for metastatic disease. PD-L1 status was determined using the PD-L1 IHC 22C3 pharmDx™ kit. Patients with an autoimmune disease that required systemic therapy within 2 years of treatment or a medical condition that required immunosuppression were ineligible. Randomization was stratified by PD-L1 expression (CPS ≥1 or CPS <1), chemotherapy regimen (5-FU plus cisplatin [FP] or capecitabine plus oxaliplatin [CAPOX]), and geographic region (Europe/Israel/North America/Australia, Asia, or Rest of the World). Patients were randomized (1:1) to one of the following treatment arms:

• KEYTRUDA 200 mg, trastuzumab 8 mg/kg on first infusion and 6 mg/kg in subsequent cycles, followed by investigator's choice of combination chemotherapy of cisplatin 80 mg/m^2 for up to 6 cycles and 5-FU 800 mg/m^2/day for 5 days (FP) or oxaliplatin 130 mg/m^2 up to 6-8 cycles and capecitabine 1000 mg/m^2 bid for 14 days (CAPOX). KEYTRUDA was administered prior to trastuzumab and chemotherapy on Day 1 of each cycle.

• Placebo,trastuzumab 8 mg/kg on first infusion and 6 mg/kg in subsequent cycles, followed by investigator's choice of combination chemotherapy of cisplatin 80 mg/m^2 for up to 6 cycles and 5-FU 800 mg/m^2/day for 5 days (FP) or oxaliplatin 130 mg/m^2 up to 6-8 cycles and capecitabine 1000 mg/m^2 bid for 14 days (CAPOX). All study medications, except oral capecitabine, were administered as an intravenous infusion every 3-week cycle. Treatment with KEYTRUDA continued until RECIST v1.1-defined progression of disease as determined by BICR, unacceptable toxicity, or a maximum of 24 months.

In an interim efficacy analysis, the major outcome measures assessed were ORR and DoR by BICR using RECIST v1.1, modified to follow a maximum of 10 target lesions and a maximum of 5 target lesions per organ.

At the time of the interim analysis, ORR and DoR were assessed in the first 264 patients randomized. Among the 264 patients, the population characteristics were: median age of 62 years (range: 19 to 84), 41% age 65 or older; 82% male; 63% White, 31% Asian, and 0.8% Black; 47% ECOG PS of 0 and 53% ECOG PS of 1. Ninety-seven percent of patients had metastatic disease (Stage IV) and 3% had locally advanced unresectable disease. Ninety-one percent (n=240) had tumors that were not MSI-H, 1% (n=2) had tumors that were MSI-H, and in 8% (n=22) the status was not known. Eighty-seven percent of patients received CAPOX.

A statistically significant improvement in ORR was demonstrated in patients randomized to KEYTRUDA in combination with trastuzumab and chemotherapy compared with placebo in combination with trastuzumab and chemotherapy.

14.11. Esophageal Cancer First-line Treatment of Locally Advanced Unresectable or Metastatic Esophageal/Gastroesophageal Junction Cancer

The efficacy of KEYTRUDA was investigated in KEYNOTE-590 (NCT03189719), a multicenter, randomized, placebo-controlled trial that enrolled 749 patients with metastatic or locally advanced esophageal or gastroesophageal junction (tumors with epicenter 1 to 5 centimeters above the GEJ) carcinoma who were not candidates for surgical resection or definitive chemoradiation. PD-L1 status was centrally determined in tumor specimens in all patients using the PD-L1 IHC 22C3 pharmDx kit. Patients with active autoimmune disease, a medical condition that required immunosuppression, or who received prior systemic therapy in the locally advanced or metastatic setting were ineligible. Randomization was stratified by tumor histology (squamous cell carcinoma vs. adenocarcinoma), geographic region (Asia vs. ex-Asia), and ECOG performance status (0 vs. 1). Patients were randomized (1:1) to one of the following treatment arms; all study medications were administered via intravenous infusion:

• KEYTRUDA 200 mg on Day 1 of each three-week cycle in combination with cisplatin 80 mg/m^2 IV on Day 1 of each three-week cycle for up to six cycles and FU 800 mg/m^2 IV per day on Day 1 to Day 5 of each three-week cycle, or per local standard for FU administration, for up to 24 months.

• Placebo on Day 1 of each three-week cycle in combination with cisplatin 80 mg/m^2 IV on Day 1 of each three-week cycle for up to six cycles and FU 800 mg/m^2 IV per day on Day 1 to Day 5 of each three-week cycle, or per local standard for FU administration, for up to 24 months. Treatment with KEYTRUDA or chemotherapy continued until unacceptable toxicity or disease progression. Patients could be treated with KEYTRUDA for up to 24 months in the absence of disease progression. The major efficacy outcome measures were OS and PFS as assessed by the investigator according to RECIST v1.1 (modified to follow a maximum of 10 target lesions and a maximum of 5 target lesions per organ). The study pre-specified analyses of OS and PFS based on squamous cell histology, CPS ≥10, and in all patients. Additional efficacy outcome measures were ORR and DoR, according to modified RECIST v1.1, as assessed by the investigator.

The study population characteristics were: median age of 63 years (range: 27 to 94), 43% age 65 or older; 83% male; 37% White, 53% Asian, and 1% Black; 40% had an ECOG PS of 0 and 60% had an ECOG PS of 1. Ninety-one percent had M1 disease and 9% had M0 disease. Seventy-three percent had a tumor histology of squamous cell carcinoma, and 27% had adenocarcinoma.

The trial demonstrated a statistically significant improvement in OS and PFS for patients randomized to KEYTRUDA in combination with chemotherapy, compared to chemotherapy.

Previously Treated Recurrent Locally Advanced or Metastatic Esophageal Cancer

The efficacy of KEYTRUDA was investigated in KEYNOTE-181 (NCT02564263), a multicenter, randomized, open-label, active-controlled trial that enrolled 628 patients with recurrent locally advanced or metastatic esophageal cancer who progressed on or after one prior line of systemic treatment for advanced disease. Patients with HER2/neu positive esophageal cancer were required to have received treatment with approved HER2/neu targeted therapy. All patients were required to have tumor specimens for PD-L1 testing at a central laboratory; PD-L1 status was determined using the PD-L1 IHC 22C3 pharmDx kit. Patients with a history of non-infectious pneumonitis that required steroids or current pneumonitis, active autoimmune disease, or a medical condition that required immunosuppression were ineligible.

Patients were randomized (1:1) to receive either KEYTRUDA 200 mg every 3 weeks or investigator's choice of any of the following chemotherapy regimens, all given intravenously: paclitaxel 80-100 mg/m^2 on Days 1, 8, and 15 of every 4-week cycle, docetaxel 75 mg/m^2 every 3 weeks, or irinotecan 180 mg/m^2 every 2 weeks. Randomization was stratified by tumor histology (esophageal squamous cell carcinoma [ESCC] vs. esophageal adenocarcinoma [EAC]/Siewert type I EAC of the gastroesophageal junction [GEJ]), and geographic region (Asia vs. ex-Asia).

Treatment with KEYTRUDA or chemotherapy continued until unacceptable toxicity or disease progression. Patients randomized to KEYTRUDA were permitted to continue beyond the first RECIST v1.1 (modified to follow a maximum of 10 target lesions and a maximum of 5 target lesions per organ)-defined disease progression if clinically stable until the first radiographic evidence of disease progression was confirmed at least 4 weeks later with repeat imaging. Patients treated with KEYTRUDA without disease progression could be treated for up to 24 months. Assessment of tumor status was performed every 9 weeks.

The major efficacy outcome measure was OS evaluated in the following co-primary populations: patients with ESCC, patients with tumors expressing PD-L1 CPS ≥10, and all randomized patients. Additional efficacy outcome measures were PFS, ORR, and DoR, according to RECIST v1.1, modified to follow a maximum of 10 target lesions and a maximum of 5 target lesions per organ, as assessed by BICR. A total of 628 patients were enrolled and randomized to KEYTRUDA (n=314) or investigator's treatment of choice (n=314). Of these 628 patients, 167 (27%) had ESCC that expressed PD-L1 with a CPS ≥10. Of these 167 patients, 85 patients were randomized to KEYTRUDA and 82 patients to investigator's treatment of choice [paclitaxel (n=50), docetaxel (n=19), or irinotecan (n=13)]. The baseline characteristics of these 167 patients were: median age of 65 years (range: 33 to 80), 51% age 65 or older; 84% male; 32% White and 68% Asian; 38% had an ECOG PS of 0 and 62% had an ECOG PS of 1. Ninety percent had M1 disease and 10% had M0 disease. Prior to enrollment, 99% of patients had received platinum-based treatment and 84% had also received treatment with a fluoropyrimidine. Thirty-three percent of patients received prior treatment with a taxane.

The observed OS hazard ratio was 0.77 (95% CI: 0.63, 0.96) in patients with ESCC, 0.70 (95% CI: 0.52, 0.94) in patients with tumors expressing PD-L1 CPS ≥10, and 0.89 (95% CI: 0.75, 1.05) in all randomized patients.

On further examination in patients whose ESCC tumors expressed PD-L1 (CPS ≥10), an improvement in OS was observed among patients randomized to KEYTRUDA as compared with chemotherapy.

Locally advanced or metastatic esophageal cancer who progressed on or after at least 2 prior systemic treatments for advanced disease.

The efficacy of KEYTRUDA was investigated in KEYNOTE-180 (NCT02559687), a multicenter, nonrandomized, open-label trial that enrolled 121 patients. With the exception of the number of prior lines of treatment, the eligibility criteria were similar to, and the dosage regimen identical, to KEYNOTE-181. The major efficacy outcome measures were ORR and DoR according to RECIST v1.1, modified to follow a maximum of 10 target lesions and a maximum of 5 target lesions per organ, as assessed by BICR. Among the 121 patients enrolled, 29% (n=35) had ESCC that expressed PD-L1 CPS ≥10. The baseline characteristics of these 35 patients were: median age of 65 years (range: 47 to 81), 51% age 65 or older; 71% male; 26% White and 69% Asian; 40% had an ECOG PS of 0 and 60% had an ECOG PS of 1. One hundred percent had M1 disease.

The ORR in the 35 patients with ESCC expressing PD-L1 was 20% (95% CI: 8, 37). Among the 7 responding patients, the DoR ranged from 4.2 to 25.1+ months, with 5 patients (71%) having responses of 6 months or longer and 3 patients (57%) having responses of 12 months or longer.

14.12. Cervical Cancer FIGO 2014 Stage III-IVA Cervical Cancer with Chemoradiotherapy

The efficacy of KEYTRUDA in combination with CRT (cisplatin and external beam radiation therapy [EBRT] followed by brachytherapy [BT]) was investigated in KEYNOTE-A18 (NCT04221945), a multicenter, randomized, double-blind, placebo-controlled trial that enrolled 1060 patients with cervical cancer who had not previously received any definitive surgery, radiation, or systemic therapy for cervical cancer. There were 596 patients with FIGO 2014 Stage III-IVA (tumor involvement of the lower vagina with or without extension onto pelvic sidewall or hydronephrosis/non-functioning kidney or has spread to adjacent pelvic organs) with either node-positive or node-negative disease, and 462 patients with FIGO 2014 Stage IB2-IIB (tumor lesions >4 cm or clinically visible lesions that have spread beyond the uterus but have not extended onto the pelvic wall or to the lower third of vagina) with node-positive disease; two patients had FIGO 2014 Stage IVB disease.

Randomization was stratified by planned type of EBRT (Intensity-modulated radiation therapy [IMRT] or volumetric modulated arc therapy [VMAT] vs. non-IMRT and non-VMAT), stage at screening of cervical cancer (FIGO 2014 Stage IB2-IIB vs. FIGO 2014 Stage III-IVA), and planned total radiotherapy dose (EBRT + brachytherapy dose of <70 Gy vs. ≥70 Gy as per equivalent dose [EQD2]).

Patients were randomized (1:1) to one of two treatment arms:

- KEYTRUDA 200 mg IV every 3 weeks (5 cycles) concurrent with cisplatin 40 mg/m^2 IV weekly (5 cycles, an optional sixth infusion could be administered per local practice), and radiotherapy (EBRT followed by BT), followed by KEYTRUDA 400 mg IV every 6 weeks (15 cycles)

- Placebo IV every 3 weeks (5 cycles) concurrent with cisplatin 40 mg/m2 IV weekly (5 cycles, an optional sixth infusion could be administered per local practice), and radiotherapy (EBRT followed by BT), followed by placebo IV every 6 weeks (15 cycles) Treatment continued until RECIST v1.1-defined progression of disease as determined by investigator or unacceptable toxicity. Assessment of tumor status was performed every 12 weeks from completion of CRT for the first two years, followed by every 24 weeks in year 3, and then annually.

The major efficacy outcome measures were PFS as assessed by investigator according to RECIST v1.1, modified to follow a maximum of 10 target lesions and a maximum of 5 target lesions per organ, or histopathologic confirmation, and OS.

Among the 596 patients with FIGO 2014 Stage III-IVA disease, the baseline characteristics were: median age of 52 years (range: 22 to 87), 17% age 65 or older; 36% White, 34% Asian, 1% Black; 38% Hispanic or Latino; 68% ECOG PS 0 and 32% ECOG PS 1; 93% with CPS ≥1; 70% had positive pelvic and/or positive para-aortic lymph node(s) and 30% had neither positive pelvic nor para-aortic lymph node(s); 83% had squamous cell carcinoma and 17% had non-squamous histology. Regarding radiation, 85% of patients received IMRT or VMAT EBRT, and the median EQD2 dose was 87 Gy (range: 7 to 114).

The trial demonstrated a statistically significant improvement in PFS in the overall population. In an exploratory subgroup analysis for the 462 patients (44%) with FIGO 2014 Stage IB2-IIB disease, the PFS HR estimate was 0.91 (95% CI: 0.63, 1.31), indicating that the PFS improvement in the overall population was primarily attributed to the results seen in the subgroup of patients with FIGO 2014 Stage III-IVA disease. OS data were not mature at the time of PFS analysis, with 10% deaths in the overall population.

Persistent, Recurrent, or Metastatic Cervical Cancer

The efficacy of KEYTRUDA in combination with paclitaxel and cisplatin or paclitaxel and carboplatin, with or without bevacizumab, was investigated in KEYNOTE-826 (NCT03635567), a multicenter, randomized, double-blind, placebo-controlled trial that enrolled 617 patients with persistent, recurrent, or first-line metastatic cervical cancer who had not been treated with chemotherapy except when used concurrently as a radio-sensitizing agent.

Patients were enrolled regardless of tumor PD-L1 expression status. Patients with autoimmune disease that required systemic therapy within 2 years of treatment or a medical condition that required immunosuppression were ineligible. Randomization was stratified by metastatic status at initial diagnosis, investigator decision to use bevacizumab, and PD-L1 status (CPS <1% vs. CPS 1 to <10 vs. CPS ≥10).

Patients were randomized (1:1) to one of the two treatment groups:

• Treatment Group 1: KEYTRUDA 200 mg plus chemotherapy with or without bevacizumab

• Treatment Group 2: Placebo plus chemotherapy with or without bevacizumab The investigator selected one of the following four treatment regimens prior to randomization:

1. Paclitaxel 175 mg/m^2 + cisplatin 50 mg/m^2

2. Paclitaxel 175 mg/m^2 + cisplatin 50 mg/m^2 + bevacizumab 15 mg/kg

3. Paclitaxel 175 mg/m^2 + carboplatin AUC 5 mg/mL/min

4. Paclitaxel 175 mg/m^2 + carboplatin AUC 5 mg/mL/min + bevacizumab 15 mg/kg

All study medications were administered as an intravenous infusion. All study treatments were administered on Day 1 of each 3-week treatment cycle. Cisplatin could be administered on Day 2 of each 3-week treatment cycle. Treatment with KEYTRUDA continued until RECIST v1.1-defined progression of disease, unacceptable toxicity, or a maximum of 24 months. Administration of KEYTRUDA was permitted beyond RECIST-defined disease progression if the patient was clinically stable and considered to be deriving clinical benefit by the investigator. Assessment of tumor status was performed every 9 weeks for the first year, followed by every 12 weeks thereafter.

The main efficacy outcome measures were OS and PFS as assessed by investigator according to RECIST v1.1, modified to follow a maximum of 10 target lesions and a maximum of 5 target lesions per organ. Additional efficacy outcome measures were ORR and DoR, according to RECIST v1.1, as assessed by investigator. Of the 617 enrolled patients, 548 patients (89%) had tumors expressing PD-L1 with a CPS ≥1. Among these 548 enrolled patients with tumors expressing PD-L1, 273 patients were randomized to KEYTRUDA in combination with chemotherapy with or without bevacizumab, and 275 patients were randomized to placebo in combination with chemotherapy with or without bevacizumab. Sixty-three percent of the 548 patients received bevacizumab as part of study treatment.

The baseline characteristics of the 548 patients were: median age of 51 years (range: 22 to 82), 16% age 65 or older; 59% White, 18% Asian, 6% American Indian or Alaska Native, and 1% Black; 37% Hispanic or Latino; 56% ECOG performance status 0 and 43% ECOG performance status 1. Seventy-five percent had squamous cell carcinoma, 21% adenocarcinoma, and 5% adenosquamous histology, and 32% of patients had metastatic disease at diagnosis. At study entry, 21% of patients had metastatic disease only and 79% had persistent or recurrent disease with or without distant metastases, of whom 39% had received prior chemoradiation only and 17% had received prior chemoradiation plus surgery.

A statistically significant improvement in OS and PFS was demonstrated in patients randomized to receive KEYTRUDA compared with patients randomized to receive placebo.

Previously Treated Recurrent or Metastatic Cervical Cancer

The efficacy of KEYTRUDA was investigated in 98 patients with recurrent or metastatic cervical cancer enrolled in a single cohort (Cohort E) in KEYNOTE-158 (NCT02628067), a multicenter, non-randomized, open-label, multi-cohort trial. The trial excluded patients with autoimmune disease or a medical condition that required immunosuppression.

Patients received KEYTRUDA 200 mg intravenously every 3 weeks until unacceptable toxicity or documented disease progression. Patients with initial radiographic disease progression could receive additional doses of treatment during confirmation of progression unless disease progression was symptomatic, was rapidly progressive, required urgent intervention, or occurred with a decline in performance status. Patients without disease progression could be treated for up to 24 months. Assessment of tumor status was performed every 9 weeks for the first 12 months, and every 12 weeks thereafter.

The major efficacy outcome measures were ORR according to RECIST v1.1, modified to follow a maximum of 10 target lesions and a maximum of 5 target lesions per organ, as assessed by BICR, and DoR. Among the 98 patients in Cohort E, 77

(79%) had tumors that expressed PD-L1 with a CPS ≥ 1 and received at least one line of chemotherapy in the metastatic setting. PD-L1 status was determined using the IHC 22C3 pharmDx kit. The baseline characteristics of these 77 patients were: median age of 45 years (range: 27 to 75); 81% White, 14% Asian, and 3% Black; 32% ECOG PS of 0 and 68% ECOG PS of 1; 92% had squamous cell carcinoma, 6% adenocarcinoma, and 1% adeno-squamous histology; 95% had M1 disease and 5% had recurrent disease; and 35% had one and 65% had two or more prior lines of therapy in the recurrent or metastatic setting.

No responses were observed in patients whose tumors did not have PD-L1 expression (CPS <1).

14.13 Hepatocellular Carcinoma (HCC)

The efficacy of KEYTRUDA was investigated in KEYNOTE-394 (NCT03062358), a multicenter, randomized, placebo-controlled, double-blind trial conducted in Asia in patients with Barcelona Clinic Liver Cancer (BCLC) Stage B or C HCC, who were previously treated with sorafenib or oxaliplatin-based chemotherapy and who were not amenable to or were refractory to local-regional therapy. Patients were also required to have Child-Pugh A liver function. Patients with hepatitis B had treated controlled disease (HBV viral load <2000 IU/ml or $<10^4$ copies/ml). Patients with an autoimmune disease that required systemic therapy within 2 years of treatment or a medical condition that required immunosuppression were ineligible. Patients with hepatic encephalopathy, main branch portal venous invasion, clinically apparent ascites, or esophageal or gastric variceal bleeding within the last 6 months were also ineligible.

Randomization was stratified by prior treatment: sorafenib vs. oxaliplatin-based chemotherapy, macrovascular invasion, and etiology (active HBV vs. others (active HCV, non-infected)). Patients were randomized (2:1) to receive pembrolizumab 200 mg intravenously every 3 weeks or placebo. Treatment with KEYTRUDA continued until RECIST v1.1-defined progression of disease as determined by BICR, unacceptable toxicity, or a maximum of 24 months. Assessment of tumor status was performed every 6 weeks.

The main efficacy outcome measure was OS. Additional efficacy outcome measures were PFS, ORR, and DoR, as assessed by BICR using RECIST v1.1, modified to follow a maximum of 10 target lesions and a maximum of 5 target lesions per organ. The study enrolled 453 patients, and 360 (79%) had active hepatitis B. The population characteristics in patients with active hepatitis B were: median age of 52 years (range: 23 to 82), 16% age 65 or older; 86% male; 100% Asian; 42% ECOG PS of 0 and 58% ECOG PS of 1; 90% received prior sorafenib and 10% received prior oxaliplatin-based chemotherapy. Patient characteristics also included extrahepatic disease (77%), macrovascular invasion (10%), BCLC stage C (93%) and B (7%), and baseline AFP ≥200 ng/mL (57%).

KEYNOTE-394 demonstrated improved OS in patients with HCC secondary to hepatitis B randomized to KEYTRUDA compared with placebo.

14.14 Biliary Tract Cancer

The efficacy of KEYTRUDA in combination with gemcitabine and cisplatin chemotherapy was investigated in KEYNOTE-966 (NCT04003636), a multicenter, randomized, double-blind, placebocontrolled trial that enrolled 1069 patients with locally advanced unresectable or metastatic BTC, who had not received prior systemic therapy in the advanced disease setting. Patients with autoimmune disease that required systemic therapy within 2 years of treatment or a medical condition that required immunosuppression were ineligible.

Randomization was stratified by region (Asia vs. non-Asia), locally advanced versus metastatic, and site of origin (gallbladder, intrahepatic or extrahepatic cholangiocarcinoma). Patients were randomized (1:1) to KEYTRUDA 200 mg on Day 1 plus gemcitabine 1000 mg/m^2 and cisplatin 25 mg/m^2 on Day 1 and Day 8 every 3 weeks, or placebo on Day 1 plus gemcitabine 1000 mg/m^2 and cisplatin 25 mg/m^2 on Day 1 and Day 8 every 3 weeks. Study medications were administered via intravenous infusion. Treatment continued until unacceptable toxicity or disease progression. For pembrolizumab, treatment continued for a maximum of 35 cycles, or approximately 24 months. For gemcitabine, treatment could be continued beyond 8 cycles while for cisplatin, treatment could be administered for a maximum of 8 cycles. Administration of KEYTRUDA with chemotherapy was permitted beyond RECIST-defined disease progression if the patient was clinically stable and considered by the investigator to be deriving clinical benefit. Assessment of tumor status was performed at baseline and then every 6 weeks through 54 weeks, followed by every 12 weeks thereafter.

Study population characteristics were median age of 64 years (range: 23 to 85), 47% age 65 or older; 52% male; 49% White, 46% Asian, 1.3% Black or African American; 10% Hispanic or Latino; 46% ECOG PS of 0 and 54% ECOG PS of 1; 31% of patients had a history of hepatitis B infection, and 3% had a history of hepatitis C infection.

The major efficacy outcome measure was OS. Additional efficacy outcome measures were PFS, ORR and DoR as assessed by BICR according to RECIST v11.1, modified to follow a maximum of 10 target lesions and a maximum of 5 target lesions per organ.

Overall survival was 78% in the KEYTRUDA group and 83% in the placebo group. The median duration of overall survival was 12.7 and 10.9 months respectively. p-value 0.0034.

14.15 Merkel Cell Carcinoma

The efficacy of KEYTRUDA was investigated in KEYNOTE-017 (NCT02267603) and KEYNOTE-913 (NCT03783078), two multicenter, non-randomized, open-label trials that enrolled 105 patients with recurrent locally advanced or metastatic MCC who had not received prior systemic therapy for their advanced disease. Patients with active autoimmune disease or a medical condition that required immunosuppression were ineligible.

Patients received KEYTRUDA 2 mg/kg (KEYNOTE-017) or 200 mg (KEYNOTE-913) every 3 weeks until unacceptable toxicity or disease progression that was symptomatic, rapidly progressive, required urgent intervention, occurred with a decline in performance status, or was confirmed at least 4 weeks later with repeat imaging. Patients without disease progression were treated for up to 24 months.

The major efficacy outcome measures were ORR and DoR as assessed by BICR per RECIST v1.1. Among the 105 patients enrolled, the median age was 73 years (range: 38 to 91), 79% were age 65 or older; 62% were male; 80% were White, race in 19% was unknown or missing, and 1% were Asian; 53% had ECOG PS of 0, and 47% had ECOG PS of 1. Thirteen percent had stage IIIB disease and 84% had stage IV. Seventy-six percent of patients had prior surgery and 51% had prior radiation therapy.

The objective response rates in the two trials were 56% and 49% respectively. The median duration (months) was not reached in either trial.

14.16 Renal Cell Carcinoma

The efficacy of KEYTRUDA in combination with axitinib was investigated in KEYNOTE-426 (NCT02853331), a randomized, multicenter, open-label trial conducted in 861 patients who had not received systemic therapy for advanced RCC. Patients were enrolled regardless of PD-L1 tumor expression status. Patients with active autoimmune disease requiring systemic immunosuppression within the last 2 years were ineligible.

Randomization was stratified by International Metastatic RCC Database Consortium (IMDC) risk categories (favorable versus intermediate versus poor) and geographic region (North America versus Western Europe versus Rest of the World). Patients were randomized (1:1) to one of the following treatment arms:

• KEYTRUDA 200 mg intravenously every 3 weeks up to 24 months in combination with axitinib 5 mg orally, twice daily. Patients who tolerated axitinib 5 mg twice daily for 2 consecutive cycles (6 weeks) could increase to 7 mg and then subsequently to 10 mg twice daily. Axitinib could be interrupted or reduced to 3 mg twice daily and subsequently to 2 mg twice daily to manage toxicity.

• Sunitinib 50 mg orally, once daily for 4 weeks and then off treatment for 2 weeks. Treatment with KEYTRUDA and axitinib continued until RECIST v1.1-defined progression of disease or unacceptable toxicity. Administration of KEYTRUDA and axitinib was permitted beyond RECIST-defined disease progression if the patient was clinically stable and considered to be deriving clinical benefit by the investigator. Assessment of tumor status was performed at baseline, after randomization at Week 12, then every 6 weeks thereafter until Week 54, and then every 12 weeks thereafter.

The study population characteristics were: median age of 62 years (range: 26 to 90), 38% age 65 or older; 73% male; 79% White and 16% Asian; 20% and 80% of patients had a baseline KPS of 70 to 80 and 90 to 100, respectively; and patient distribution by IMDC risk categories was 31% favorable, 56% intermediate, and 13% poor.

The main efficacy outcome measures were OS and PFS as assessed by BICR according to RECIST v1.1, modified to follow a maximum of 10 target lesions and a maximum of 5 target lesions per organ. Additional efficacy outcome measures included ORR, as assessed by BICR.

A statistically significant improvement in OS was demonstrated at the first pre-specified interim analysis in patients randomized to KEYTRUDA in combination with axitinib compared with sunitinib. The trial also demonstrated statistically significant improvements in PFS and ORR.

First-line treatment with lenvatinib

The efficacy of KEYTRUDA in combination with lenvatinib was investigated in KEYNOTE-581 (NCT02811861), a multicenter, open-label, randomized trial conducted in 1069 patients with advanced RCC in the first-line setting. Patients were enrolled regardless of PD-L1 tumor expression status. Patients with active autoimmune disease or a medical condition that required immunosuppression were ineligible. Randomization was stratified by geographic region (North America versus Western Europe versus Rest of the World) and Memorial Sloan Kettering Cancer Center (MSKCC) prognostic groups (favorable versus intermediate versus poor risk).

Patients were randomized (1:1:1) to one of the following treatment arms:

• KEYTRUDA 200 mg intravenously every 3 weeks up to 24 months in combination with lenvatinib 20 mg orally once daily.

• Lenvatinib 18 mg orally once daily in combination with everolimus 5 mg orally once daily.

• Sunitinib 50 mg orally once daily for 4 weeks then off treatment for 2 weeks.

Treatment continued until unacceptable toxicity or disease progression. Administration of KEYTRUDA with lenvatinib was permitted beyond RECIST-defined disease progression if the patient was clinically stable and considered by the investigator to be deriving clinical benefit. KEYTRUDA was continued for a maximum of 24 months; however, treatment with lenvatinib could be continued beyond 24 months. Assessment of tumor status was performed at baseline and then every 8 weeks.

The study population characteristics were: median age of 62 years (range: 29 to 88 years), 42% age 65 or older; 75% male; 74% White, 21% Asian, 1% Black, and 2% other races; 18% and 82% of patients had a baseline KPS of 70 to 80 and 90 to 100, respectively; patient distribution by MSKCC risk categories was 27% favorable, 64% intermediate, and 9% poor. Common sites of metastases in patients were lung (68%), lymph node (45%), and bone (25%).

The major efficacy outcome measures were PFS, as assessed by independent radiologic review (IRC) according to RECIST v1.1, and OS. Additional efficacy outcome measures included confirmed ORR as assessed by IRC.

KEYTRUDA in combination with lenvatinib demonstrated statistically significant improvements in PFS, OS, and ORR compared with sunitinib.

The efficacy of KEYTRUDA in combination with lenvatinib was investigated in KEYNOTE-B61 (NCT04704219), a multicenter, single-arm trial that enrolled 160 patients with advanced or metastatic non-clear cell RCC in the first-line setting. Patients with active autoimmune disease or a medical condition that required immunosuppression were ineligible.

Patients received KEYTRUDA 400 mg every 6 weeks in combination with lenvatinib 20 mg orally once daily. KEYTRUDA was continued for a maximum of 24 months; however, lenvatinib could be continued beyond 24 months. Treatment continued until unacceptable toxicity or disease progression. Administration of KEYTRUDA with lenvatinib was permitted beyond RECIST-defined disease progression if the patient was considered by the investigator to be deriving clinical benefit.

Among the 158 treated patients, the baseline characteristics were: median age of 60 years (range: 24 to 87 years); 71% male; 86% White, 8% Asian, and 3% Black; <1% Hispanic or Latino; 22% and 78% of patients had a baseline KPS of 70 to 80 and 90 to 100, respectively; histologic subtypes were 59% papillary, 18% chromophobe, 4% translocation, <1% medullary, 13% unclassified, and 6% other; patient distribution by IMDC risk categories was 35% favorable, 54% intermediate, and 10% poor.

Common sites of metastases in patients were lymph node (65%), lung (35%), bone (30%), and liver (21%).

The major efficacy outcome measure was ORR as assessed by BICR using RECIST 1.1. Additional efficacy outcome measures included DOR as assessed by BICR using RECIST 1.1.

The objective response rate was 51% and the median duration of response was 19.5 months.

Adjuvant Treatment of RCC

The efficacy of KEYTRUDA was investigated as adjuvant therapy for RCC in KEYNOTE-564 (NCT03142334), a multicenter, randomized (1:1), double-blind, placebo-controlled trial in 994 patients with intermediate-high or high risk of recurrence of RCC, or M1 no evidence of disease (NED). The intermediate-high risk category included: pT2 with Grade 4 or sarcomatoid features; pT3, any Grade without nodal involvement (N0) or distant metastases (M0). The high risk category included: pT4, any Grade N0 and M0; any pT, any Grade with nodal involvement and M0. The M1 NED category included patients with metastatic disease who had undergone complete resection of primary and metastatic lesions.

Patients must have undergone a partial nephroprotective or radical complete nephrectomy (and complete resection of solid, isolated, soft tissue metastatic lesion(s) in M1 NED participants) with negative surgical margins ≥4 weeks prior to the time of screening. Patients were excluded from the trial if they had received prior systemic therapy for advanced RCC. Patients with active autoimmune disease or a medical condition that required immunosuppression were also ineligible.

Patients were randomized to KEYTRUDA 200 mg administered intravenously every 3 weeks or placebo for up to 1 year until disease recurrence or unacceptable toxicity. Randomization was stratified by metastasis status (M0, M1 NED); M0 group was further stratified by ECOG PS (0,1) and geographic region (US, non-US).

The study population characteristics were: median age of 60 years (range: 25 to 84), 33% age 65 or older; 71% male; 75% White, 14% Asian, 9% Unknown, 1% Black or African American, 1% American Indian or Alaska Native, 1% Multiracial; 13% Hispanic or Latino, 78% Not Hispanic or Latino, 8% Unknown; and 85% ECOG PS of

0 and 15% ECOG PS of 1. Ninety-four percent of patients enrolled had N0 disease; 11% had sarcomatoid features; 86% were intermediate-high risk; 8% were high risk; and 6% were M1 NED. Ninety-two percent of patients had a radical nephrectomy, and 8% had a partial nephrectomy.

The major efficacy outcome measure was investigator-assessed disease-free survival (DFS), defined as time to recurrence, metastasis, or death. An additional outcome measure was OS.

Statistically significant improvements in DFS and OS were demonstrated at pre-specified interim analyses in patients randomized to the KEYTRUDA arm compared with placebo.

14.17 Endometrial Carcinoma In Combination with Paclitaxel and Carboplatin for the Treatment of Primary Advanced or Recurrent Endometrial Carcinoma

The efficacy of KEYTRUDA in combination with paclitaxel and carboplatin was investigated in KEYNOTE-868/NRG-GY018 (NCT03914612), a multicenter, randomized, double-blind, placebo-controlled trial in 810 patients with advanced or recurrent endometrial carcinoma. The study design included two separate cohorts based on MMR status; 222 (27%) patients were in dMMR cohort, 588 (73%) patients were in pMMR cohort. The trial enrolled measurable Stage III, measurable Stage IVA, Stage IVB or recurrent endometrial cancer (with or without measurable disease). Patients who had not received prior systemic therapy or had received prior chemotherapy in the adjuvant setting were eligible. Patients who had received prior adjuvant chemotherapy were only eligible if their chemotherapy-free interval was at least 12 months. Patients with endometrial sarcoma, including carcinosarcoma, or patients with active autoimmune disease or a medical condition that required immunosuppression were ineligible. Randomization was stratified according to MMR status, ECOG PS (0 or 1 vs. 2), and prior adjuvant chemotherapy. Patients were randomized (1:1) to one of the following treatment arms:

• KEYTRUDA 200 mg every 3 weeks, paclitaxel 175 mg/m^2 and carboplatin AUC 5 mg/mL/min for 6 cycles, followed by KEYTRUDA 400 mg every 6 weeks for up to 14 cycles.

• Placebo every 3 weeks, paclitaxel 175 mg/m^2 and carboplatin AUC 5 mg/mL/min for 6 cycles, followed by placebo every 6 weeks for up to 14 cycles. All study medications were administered as an intravenous infusion on Day 1 of each treatment cycle. Treatment continued until disease progression, unacceptable toxicity, or a maximum of 20 cycles (up to approximately 24 months). Patients with measurable disease who had RECIST-defined stable disease or partial response at the completion of cycle 6 were permitted to continue receiving paclitaxel and carboplatin with KEYTRUDA or placebo for up to 10 cycles as determined by the investigator. Assessment of tumor status was performed every 9 weeks for the first 9 months and then every 12 weeks thereafter.

The major efficacy outcome measure was PFS as assessed by the investigator according to RECIST 1.1. An additional efficacy outcome measure was OS. The dMMR population characteristics were: median age of 66 years (range: 37 to 86), 55% age 65 or older; 79% White, 9% Black, and 3% Asian; 5% Hispanic or Latino; 64% ECOG PS of 0, 33% ECOG PS of 1, and 3% ECOG PS of 2; 61% had recurrent disease and 39% had primary or persistent disease; 5% received prior adjuvant chemotherapy and 43% received prior radiotherapy. The histologic subtypes were endometrioid carcinoma (81%), adenocarcinoma NOS (11%), serous carcinoma (2%), and other (6%). The pMMR population characteristics were: median age of 66 years (range: 29 to 94), 54% age 65 or older; 72% White, 16% Black, and 5% Asian; 6% Hispanic or Latino; 67% ECOG PS of 0, 30% ECOG PS of 1, and 3% ECOG PS of 2; 56% had recurrent disease and 44% had primary or persistent disease; 26% received prior adjuvant chemotherapy and 41% received prior radiotherapy. The histologic subtypes were endometrioid carcinoma (52%), serous carcinoma (26%), adenocarcinoma NOS (10%), clear cell carcinoma (7%), and other (5%).

The trial demonstrated statistically significant improvements in PFS for patients randomized to KEYTRUDA in combination with paclitaxel and carboplatin compared to placebo in combination with paclitaxel and carboplatin in both the dMMR and pMMR populations.

In Combination with Lenvatinib for the Treatment of Advanced Endometrial Carcinoma that Is pMMR or Not MSI-H

The efficacy of KEYTRUDA in combination with lenvatinib was investigated in KEYNOTE-775 (NCT03517449), a multicenter, open-label, randomized, active-controlled trial that enrolled 827 patients with advanced endometrial carcinoma who had been previously treated with at least one prior platinum-based chemotherapy regimen in any setting, including in the neoadjuvant and adjuvant settings. Patients with endometrial sarcoma, including carcinosarcoma, or patients who had active autoimmune disease or a medical condition that required immunosuppression were ineligible.

Patients with endometrial carcinoma that were pMMR (using the VENTANA MMR RxDx Panel test) or not MSI-H were stratified by ECOG performance status, geographic region, and history of pelvic radiation. Patients were randomized (1:1) to one of the following treatment arms:

• KEYTRUDA 200 mg intravenously every 3 weeks in combination with lenvatinib 20 mg orally once daily.

• Investigator's choice, consisting of either doxorubicin 60 mg/m^2 every 3 weeks or paclitaxel 80 mg/m^2 given weekly, 3 weeks on/1 week off.

Treatment with KEYTRUDA and lenvatinib continued until RECIST v1.1-defined progression of disease as verified by BICR, unacceptable toxicity, or for KEYTRUDA, a maximum of 24 months. Treatment was permitted beyond RECIST v1.1-defined disease progression if the treating investigator considered the patient to be deriving clinical benefit, and the treatment was tolerated. Assessment of tumor status was performed every 8 weeks.

The major efficacy outcome measures were OS and PFS as assessed by BICR according to RECIST v1.1, modified to follow a maximum of 10 target lesions and a maximum of 5 target lesions per organ. Additional efficacy outcome measures included ORR and DoR, as assessed by BICR. Among the 697 pMMR patients, 346 patients were randomized to KEYTRUDA in combination with lenvatinib, and 351 patients were randomized to investigator's choice of doxorubicin (n=254) or paclitaxel (n=97).

The pMMR population characteristics were: median age of 65 years (range: 30 to 86), 52% age 65 or older; 62% White, 22% Asian, and 3% Black; 60% ECOG PS of 0 and 40% ECOG PS of 1. The histologic subtypes were endometrioid carcinoma (55%), serous (30%), clear cell carcinoma (7%), mixed (4%), and other (3%). All 697 of these patients received prior systemic therapy for endometrial carcinoma: 67% had one, 30% had two, and 3% had three or more prior systemic therapies. Thirty-seven percent of patients received only prior neoadjuvant or adjuvant therapy.

Overall survival was 48% andc58% in the KEYTRUDA and Lenvatinib group vs. the doxorubicin or pactitaxel groups respectively. The median survival in months was 17.4 vs. 12.o. Hazard ratio 0.68. p-value 0.0001.

As a Single Agent for the Treatment of Advanced MSI-H or dMMR Endometrial Carcinoma

The efficacy of KEYTRUDA was investigated in KEYNOTE-158 (NCT02628067), a multicenter, non-randomized, open-label, multi-cohort trial. The trial enrolled 90 patients with unresectable or metastatic MSI-H or dMMR endometrial carcinoma in Cohorts D and K who received at least one dose of KEYTRUDA. MSI or MMR tumor status was determined using polymerase chain reaction (PCR) or immunohistochemistry (IHC), respectively. Patients with autoimmune disease or a medical condition that required immunosuppression were ineligible.

Patients received KEYTRUDA 200 mg intravenously every 3 weeks until unacceptable toxicity or documented disease progression. Patients treated with KEYTRUDA without disease progression could be treated for up to 24 months. Assessment of tumor status was performed every 9 weeks for the first 12 months, and every 12 weeks thereafter. The major efficacy outcome measures were ORR and DoR as assessed by BICR according to RECIST v1.1, modified to follow a maximum of 10 target lesions and a maximum of 5 target lesions per organ.

Among the 90 patients evaluated, the baseline characteristics were: median age of 64 years (range: 42 to 86); 83% White, 8% Asian, and 3% Black; 12% Hispanic or Latino; 39% ECOG PS of 0 and 61% ECOG PS of 1; 96% had M1 disease and 4% had M0 disease at study entry; and 51% had one and 48% had two or more prior lines of therapy. Nine patients received only adjuvant therapy and one patient received only neoadjuvant and adjuvant therapy before participating in the study.

The objective response rate was 46%. The median duration of response in months was not reached (range 2.9 to 55.7+).

14.18 Tumor Mutational Burden-High Cancer

The efficacy of KEYTRUDA was investigated in a prospectively-planned retrospective analysis of 10 cohorts (A through J) of patients with various previously treated unresectable or metastatic solid tumors with high tumor mutation burden (TMB-H) who were enrolled in a multicenter, non-randomized, open-label trial, KEYNOTE-158 (NCT02628067). The trial excluded patients who previously received an anti-PD-1 or other immune-modulating monoclonal antibody, or who had an autoimmune disease, or a medical condition that required immunosuppression.

Patients received KEYTRUDA 200 mg intravenously every 3 weeks until unacceptable toxicity or documented disease progression. Assessment of tumor status was performed every 9 weeks for the first 12 months and every 12 weeks thereafter. The statistical analysis plan pre-specified ≥10 and ≥13 mutations per megabase using the FoundationOne CDx assay as cutpoints to assess TMB. Testing of TMB was blinded with respect to clinical outcomes.

The major efficacy outcome measures were ORR and DoR in patients who received at least one dose of KEYTRUDA as assessed by BICR according to RECIST v1.1, modified to follow a maximum of 10 target lesions and a maximum of 5 target lesions per organ.

1050 patients were included in the efficacy analysis population. TMB was analyzed in the subset of 790 patients with sufficient tissue for testing based on protocol-specified testing requirements. Of the 790 patients, 102 (13%) had tumors identified as TMB-H, defined as TMB ≥10 mutations per megabase. Among the 102 patients with TMB-H advanced solid tumors, the study population characteristics were: median age of 61 years (range: 27 to 80), 34% age 65 or older; 34% male; 81% White; and 41% ECOG PS of 0 and 58% ECOG PS of 1. Fifty-six percent of patients had at least two prior lines of therapy.

The objective response rates in patients with TMB ≥10 mut/Mb was 29% and in those with TMB ≥13 mut/Mb it was 37%. The median duration of response in months was not reached in each group.

14.19 Cutaneous Squamous Cell Carcinoma

The efficacy of KEYTRUDA was investigated in patients with recurrent or metastatic cSCC or locally advanced cSCC enrolled in KEYNOTE-629 (NCT03284424), a multicenter, multi-cohort, non-randomized, open-label trial. The trial excluded patients with autoimmune disease or a medical condition that required immunosuppression.

Patients received KEYTRUDA 200 mg intravenously every 3 weeks until documented disease progression, unacceptable toxicity, or a maximum of 24 months. Patients with initial radiographic disease progression could receive additional doses of KEYTRUDA during confirmation of progression unless disease progression was symptomatic, rapidly progressive, required urgent intervention, or occurred with a decline in performance status. Assessment of tumor status was performed every 6 weeks during the first year, and every 9 weeks during the second year.

(Figure 46. Invasive nests with characteristic large celled centers. Ulceration (at left) is common in invasive CSCC). (

(This image is by By Mikael Häggström, M.D. Own work, CC0, https://commons.wikimedia.org/w/index.php?curid=87883012; en.wikipedia.org/wiki/Cutaneous_squamous-cell_carcinoma#/media/File:Ulcer_border_of_a_squamous_cell_skin_cancer.jpg. This file is made available under the Creative Commons CC0 1.0 Universal Public Domain Dedication. No changes were made to this image).

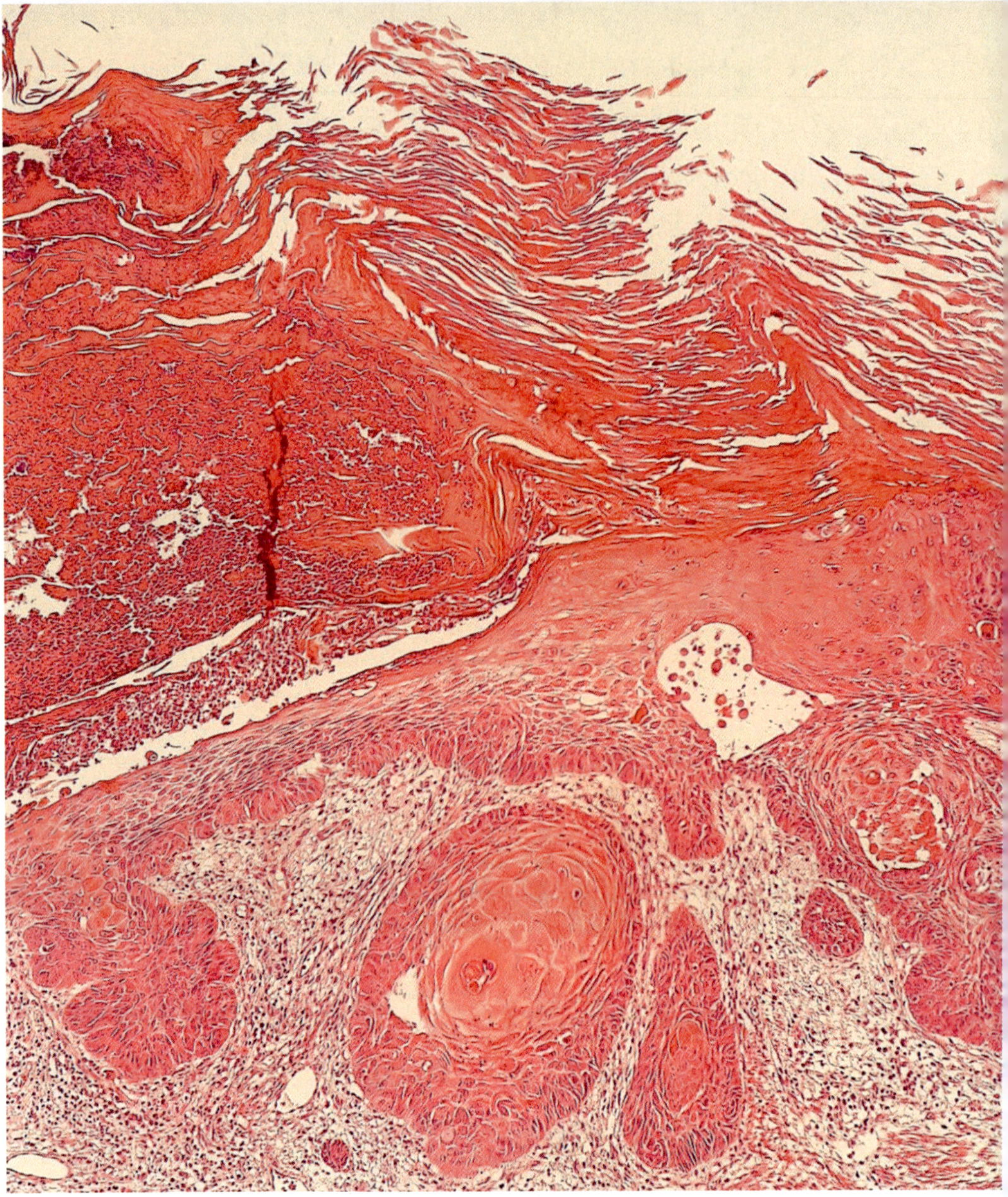

The major efficacy outcome measures were ORR and DoR as assessed by BICR according to RECIST v1.1, modified to follow a maximum of 10 target lesions and a maximum of 5 target lesions per organ. Among the 105 patients with recurrent or metastatic cSCC treated, the study population characteristics were: median age of 72 years (range: 29 to 95), 71% age 65 or older; 76% male; 71% White, 25% race unknown; 34% ECOG PS of 0 and 66% ECOG PS of 1. Forty-five percent of patients had locally recurrent only cSCC, 24% had metastatic only cSCC, and 31% had both locally recurrent and metastatic cSCC. Eighty-seven percent received one or more prior lines of therapy; 74% received prior radiation therapy.

Among the 54 patients with locally advanced cSCC treated, the study population characteristics were: median age of 76 years (range: 35 to 95), 80% age 65 or older; 72% male; 83% White, 13% race unknown; 41% ECOG PS of 0 and 59% ECOG PS of 1. Twenty-two percent received one or more prior lines of therapy; 63% received prior radiation therapy.

The objective response rate in patients with recurrent or metastatic cSCC was 35% and in those with locally advanced cSCC it was 50%. The median duration ofresponse was not reached in either group.

14.20 Triple-Negative Breast Cancer Neoadjuvant and Adjuvant Treatment of High-Risk Early-Stage TNBC

The efficacy of KEYTRUDA in combination with neoadjuvant chemotherapy followed by surgery and continued adjuvant treatment with KEYTRUDA as a single agent was investigated in KEYNOTE-522 (NCT03036488), a randomized (2:1), multicenter, double-blind, placebo-controlled trial conducted in 1174 patients with newly diagnosed previously untreated high-risk early-stage **TNBC** (tumor size >1 cm but ≤2 cm in diameter with nodal involvement or tumor size >2 cm in diameter regardless of nodal involvement).

Patients were enrolled regardless of tumor PD-L1 expression. Patients with active autoimmune disease that required systemic therapy within two years of treatment or a medical condition that required immunosuppression were ineligible. Randomization was stratified by nodal status (positive vs. negative), tumor size (T1/T2 vs. T3/T4), and choice of carboplatin (dosed every 3 weeks vs. weekly).

Patients were randomized (2:1) to one of the following two treatment arms; all study medications were administered intravenously:

Arm 1: • Four cycles of preoperative KEYTRUDA 200 mg every 3 weeks on Day 1 of cycles 1-4 of treatment regimen in combination with:

o Carboplatin AUC 5 mg/mL/min every 3 weeks on Day 1 of cycles 1-4 of treatment regimen, or AUC 1.5 mg/mL/min every week on Days 1, 8, and 15 of cycles 1-4 of treatment regimen -and

o Paclitaxel 80 mg/m^2 every week on Days 1, 8, and 15 of cycles 1-4 of treatment regimen

Followed by four additional cycles of preoperative KEYTRUDA 200 mg every 3 weeks on Day 1 of cycles 5-8 of treatment regimen in combination with:

o Doxorubicin 60 mg/m^2 or epirubicin 90 mg/m^2 every 3 weeks on Day 1 of cycles 5-8 of treatment regimen -and

o Cyclophosphamide 600 mg/m^2 every 3 weeks on Day 1 of cycles 5-8 of treatment regimen

Following surgery, nine cycles of KEYTRUDA 200 mg every 3 weeks were administered.

• Arm 2: • Four cycles of preoperative placebo every 3 weeks on Day 1 of cycles 1-4 of treatment regimen in combination with:

o Carboplatin AUC 5 mg/mL/min every 3 weeks on Day 1 of cycles 1-4 of treatment regimen or AUC 1.5 mg/mL/min every week on Days 1, 8, and 15 of cycles 1-4 of treatment regimen – and

o Paclitaxel 80 mg/m^2 every week on Days 1, 8, and 15 of cycles 1-4 of treatment regimen • Followed by four cycles of preoperative placebo every 3 weeks on Day 1 of cycles 5-8 of treatment regimen in combination with:

o Doxorubicin 60 mg/m^2 or epirubicin 90 mg/m^2 every 3 weeks on Day 1 of cycles 5-8 of treatment regimen and

o Cyclophosphamide 600 mg/m^2 every 3 weeks on Day 1 of cycles 5-8 of treatment regimen

Following surgery, nine cycles of placebo every 3 weeks were administered.

• Arm 2:

• Four cycles of preoperative placebo every 3 weeks on Day 1 of cycles 1-4 of treatment regimen in combination with:

o Carboplatin AUC 5 mg/mL/min every 3 weeks on Day 1 of cycles 1-4 of treatment regimen or AUC 1.5 mg/mL/min every week on Days 1, 8, and 15 of cycles 1-4 of treatment regimen and

o Paclitaxel 80 mg/m^2 every week on Days 1, 8, and 15 of cycles 1-4 of treatment regimen

• Followed by four cycles of preoperative placebo every 3 weeks on Day 1 of cycles 5-8 of treatment regimen in combination with:

o Doxorubicin 60 mg/m^2 or epirubicin 90 mg/m^2 every 3 weeks on Day 1 of cycles 5-8 of treatment regimen and

o Cyclophosphamide 600 mg/m^2 every 3 weeks on Day 1 of cycles 5-8 of treatment regimen

• Following surgery, nine cycles of placebo every 3 weeks were administered.

The main efficacy outcomes were pCR rate and EFS. pCR was defined as absence of invasive cancer in the breast and lymph nodes (ypT0/Tis ypN0) and was assessed by the blinded local pathologist at the time of definitive surgery. EFS was defined as the time from randomization to the first occurrence of any of the following events: progression of disease that precludes definitive surgery, local or distant recurrence, second primary malignancy, or death due to any cause. An additional efficacy outcome was overall survival (OS).

The main efficacy outcomes were pCR rate and EFS. pCR was defined as absence of invasive cancer in the breast and lymph nodes (ypT0/Tis ypN0) and was assessed by the blinded local pathologist at the time of definitive surgery. EFS was defined as the time from randomization to the first occurrence of any of the following events: progression of disease that precludes definitive surgery, local or distant recurrence, second primary malignancy, or death due to any cause. An additional efficacy outcome was overall survival (OS).

The study population characteristics were: median age of 49 years (range: 22 to 80), 11% age 65 or older; 99.9% female; 64% White, 20% Asian, 4.5% Black, and 1.8% American Indian or Alaska Native; 87% ECOG PS of 0 and 13% ECOG PS of 1; 56% were pre-menopausal status and 44% were post-menopausal status; 7% were primary tumor 1 (T1), 68% T2, 19% T3, and 7% T4; 49% were nodal involvement 0 (N0), 40% N1, 11% N2, and 0.2% N3; 75% of patients were overall Stage II and 25% were Stage III.

Event-free survival showed 16% of patients with an event in the KEYTRUDA plus chemotherapy arm vs. 23% of patients in the placebo plus chemotherapy arm, resulting a hazard ratio of 0.65 and a p value of 0.00031.

Locally Recurrent Unresectable or Metastatic TNBC

The efficacy of KEYTRUDA in combination with paclitaxel, paclitaxel protein-bound, or gemcitabine and carboplatin was investigated in KEYNOTE-355 (NCT02819518), a multicenter, double-blind, randomized, placebo-controlled trial conducted in 847 patients with locally recurrent unresectable or metastatic TNBC, regardless of tumor PD-L1 expression, who had not been previously treated with chemotherapy in the metastatic setting. Patients with active autoimmune disease that required systemic therapy within 2 years of treatment or a medical condition that required immunosuppression were ineligible.

Randomization was stratified by chemotherapy treatment (paclitaxel or paclitaxel protein-bound vs. gemcitabine and carboplatin), tumor PD-L1 expression (CPS ≥1 vs. CPS <1) according to the PD-L1 IHC 22C3 pharmDx kit, and prior treatment with the same class of chemotherapy in the neoadjuvant setting (yes vs. no).

Patients were randomized (2:1) to one of the following treatment arms; all study medications were administered via intravenous infusion:

• KEYTRUDA 200 mg on Day 1 every 3 weeks in combination with paclitaxel protein-bound 100 mg/m2 on Days 1, 8 and 15 every 28 days, paclitaxel 90 mg/m^2 on Days 1, 8, and 15 every 28 days, or gemcitabine 1000 mg/m^2 and carboplatin AUC 2 mg/mL/min on Days 1 and 8 every 21 days.

• Placebo on Day 1 every 3 weeks in combination with paclitaxel protein-bound 100 mg/m^2 on Days 1, 8 and 15 every 28 days, paclitaxel 90 mg/m^2 on Days 1, 8, and 15 every 28 days, or gemcitabine 1000 mg/m^2 and carboplatin AUC 2 mg/mL/min on Days 1 and 8 every 21 days. Assessment of tumor status was performed at Weeks 8, 16, and 24, then every 9 weeks for the first year, and every 12 weeks thereafter.

The main efficacy outcome measures were OS and PFS as assessed by BICR according to RECIST v1.1, modified to follow a maximum of 10 target lesions and a maximum of 5 target lesions per organ, tested in the subgroup of patients with CPS ≥10. Additional efficacy outcome measures were ORR and DoR as assessed by BICR. The study population characteristics for patients were: median age of 53 years (range: 22 to 85), 21% age 65 or older; 100% female; 68% White, 21% Asian, and 4% Black; 60% ECOG PS of 0 and 40% ECOG PS of 1; and 68% were post-menopausal status. Seventy-five percent of patients had tumor PD-L1 expression CPS ≥1 and 38% had tumor PD-L1 expression CPS ≥10.

The median duration in months for those patients receiving KEYTRUDA and chemotherapy was 9.7 vs, 5.6 in those receiving KEYTRUDA plus placebo, resulting a hazard ratio of 0.65 and a p-value of 0.0012.

5.4. **CEMIPRILIMAB (LIBTAYO)** HIGHLIGHTS OF PRESCRIBING INFORMATION

These highlights do not include all the information needed to use LIBTAYO safely and effectively. See full prescribing information for LIBTAYO. LIBTAYO® (cemiplimab-rwlc) injection, for intravenous use Initial U.S. Approval: 2018

INDICATIONS AND USAGE

LIBTAYO is a programmed death receptor-1 (PD-1) blocking antibody indicated in

- **Cutaneous Squamous Cell Carcinoma (CSCC)** for the treatment of patients with metastatic cutaneous squamous cell carcinoma (mCSCC) or locally advanced CSCC (laCSCC) who are not candidates for curative surgery or curative radiation
- **Basal Cell Carcinoma (BCC)** for the treatment of patients with locally advanced or metastatic BCC (laBCC or mBCC) who have been previously treated with a hedgehog pathway inhibitor or for whom a hedgehog pathway inhibitor is not appropriate
- **Non-Small Cell Lung Cancer (NSCLC)** in combination with platinum-based chemotherapy for the first-line treatment of adult patients with non-small cell lung cancer (NSCLC) with no EGFR, ALK or ROS1 aberrations and which is locally advanced where patients are not candidates for surgical resection or definitive

chemoradiation or is metastatic as a single agent for the first-line treatment of adult patients with NSCLC whose tumors have high PD-L1 expression Tumor Proportion Score (TPS) ≥ 50%] as determined by an FDA-approved test, with no EGFR, ALK or ROS1 aberrations, and is locally advanced where patients are not candidates for surgical resection or definitive chemoradiation or metastatic.

MECHANISM OF ACTION

Binding of the PD-1 ligands PD-L1 and PD-L2 to the PD-1 receptor found on T cells inhibits Tcell proliferation and cytokine production. Upregulation of PD-1 ligands occurs in some tumors and signaling through this pathway can contribute to inhibition of active T-cell immune surveillance of tumors. Cemiplimab-rwlc is a recombinant human immunoglobulin G4 (IgG4) monoclonal antibody that binds to PD-1 and blocks its interaction with PD-L1 and PD-L2, releasing PD-1 pathway-mediated inhibition of the immune response, including the anti-tumor immune response. In syngeneic mouse tumor models, blocking PD-1 activity resulted in decreased tumor growth.

DOSAGE AND ADMINISTRATION

Administer LIBTAYO as an intravenous infusion over 30 minutes after dilution. (2.2)

- CSCC and BCC: 350 mg every 3 weeks until disease progression, unacceptable toxicity, or up to 24 months.
- NSCLC: 350 mg every 3 weeks until disease progression or unacceptable toxicity

DOSAGE FORMS AND STRENGTHS Injection: 350 mg/7 mL (50 mg/mL) solution in a single-dose vial.

CONTRAINDICATIONS

None.

WARNINGS AND PRECAUTIONS

- Immune-Mediated Adverse Reactions
- Immune-mediated adverse reactions, which may be severe or fatal, can occur in any organ system or tissue, including the following: immune-mediated pneumonitis, immune-mediated colitis, immune-mediated hepatitis, immune-

mediated endocrinopathies, immune-mediated dermatologic adverse reactions, immune-mediated nephritis and renal dysfunction, and solid organ transplant rejection.

(Additional clinical details on immune-mediated adverse reactions are given in the section on nivolumab).

Monitor for early identification and management. Evaluate liver enzymes, creatinine, and thyroid function at baseline and periodically during treatment

Withhold or permanently discontinue LIBTAYO based on the severity of reaction.

- Infusion-Related Reactions

Interrupt, slow the rate of infusion, or permanently discontinue based on severity of reaction

- Complications of allogeneic hematopoietic stem cell transplantation (HSCT):

Fatal and other serious complications can occur in patients who receive allogeneic HSCT before or after being treated with a PD-1/PD-L1 blocking antibody.

- Embryo-Fetal Toxicity

Can cause fetal harm. Advise females of reproductive potential of the potential risk to a fetus and use of effective contraception.

ADVERSE REACTIONS

LIBTAYO as a Single Agent

- The most common adverse reactions (≥15%) are fatigue, musculoskeletal pain, rash, diarrhea, and anemia.

LIBTAYO in Combination with Platinum-based Chemotherapy

- The most common adverse reactions (≥15%) are alopecia, musculoskeletal pain, nausea, fatigue, peripheral neuropathy, and decreased appetite.

To report SUSPECTED ADVERSE REACTIONS, contact Regeneron at 1-877-542-3296 or FDA at 1-800-FDA-1088 or www.fda.gov/medwatch.

USE IN SPECIFIC POPULATIONS

Lactation: advise not to breastfeed.

CLINICAL STUDIES

Cutaneous Squamous Cell Carcinoma (CSCC)

The efficacy of LIBTAYO in patients with metastatic (nodal or distant) cutaneous squamous cell carcinoma (mCSCC) or locally advanced CSCC (laCSCC) who were not candidates for curative surgery or curative radiation was evaluated in two open-label, multi-center, non-randomized, multicohort studies: Study 1423 (NCT02383212) and Study 1540 (NCT02760498). Both studies excluded patients with autoimmune disease that required systemic therapy with immunosuppressant agents within 5 years; history of solid organ transplant; prior treatment with anti–PD-1/PD-L1 blocking antibodies or other immune check point inhibitor therapy; infection with HIV, hepatitis B or hepatitis C; or ECOG PS ≥ 2.

Patients received LIBTAYO 3 mg/kg intravenously every 2 weeks for up to 48 weeks in Study 1423 or up to 96 weeks (Groups 1 and 2), or 350 mg every 3 weeks for up to 54 weeks (Group 3) in Study 1540. Treatment continued until progression of disease, unacceptable toxicity, or completion of planned treatment. Tumor response assessments were performed every 8 or 9 weeks.

The major efficacy outcome measures were confirmed objective response rate (ORR), defined as complete response (CR) plus partial response (PR) as assessed by independent central review (ICR), and ICR-assessed duration of response (DOR). For patients with mCSCC without externally visible target lesions, ORR was determined by Response Evaluation Criteria in Solid Tumors (RECIST 1.1). For patients with externally visible target lesions (laCSCC and mCSCC), ORR was determined by a composite endpoint that integrated ICR assessments of radiologic data (RECIST 1.1) and digital medical photography (WHO criteria).

Study 1540

In the efficacy analysis of 193 patients with advanced CSCC enrolled in Study 1540 who received LIBTAYO at either 3 mg/kg every 2 weeks or 350 mg every three weeks, 115 had mCSCC and 78 had laCSCC. The median age was 72 years (38 to 96 years); 83% were male; 97% were White, 2% were Asian, 1% were Black or African American, and 1% were race unknown; 45% had ECOG PS 0 and 55% had ECOG PS 1; 34% received at least one prior anticancer systemic therapy; 81%

received prior cancer-related surgery; and 68% received prior radiotherapy. Among patients with mCSCC, 77% had distant metastases and 23% had only nodal metastases. For the responding patients presented in Table 10 below, the median time to response was 2.1 months (range: 1.7 to 22.8 months). Efficacy results based on the final analysis of Study 1540 are presented in Table 10.

Efficacy Endpoints	Metastatic CSCC LIBTAYO 3 mg/kg every 2 weeks (Group 1)	Locally Advanced CSCC LIBTAYO 3 mg/kg every 2 weeks (Group 2)	Metastatic CSCC LIBTAYO 350 mg every 3 weeks (Group 3)	Combined CSCC
	N = 59	N = 78	N = 56	N = 193
Confirmed Objective Response Rate (ORR) (%)				
ORR (95% CI)	51 (37, 64)	45 (34, 57)	46 (33, 60)	47 (40, 54)
Complete response rate	20	13	20	17
Partial response rate	31	32	27	30
Duration of Response (DOR)				
Number of Responders	30	35	26	91
Median DOR in months	Not reached (range 2.8 – 38.9)	42(1.9 – 54.6)	41 (4.2 – 46.3)	41(1.9 – 54.6)

Patients with observed DOR ≥ 6 months	28 (93%)	31 (89%)	25 (96%)	84 (92%)
Patients with observed DOR ≥ 12 months	23 (77%)	24 (69%)	23 (88%)	70 (77%)

Study 1423

Among 26 **CSCC** patients in Study 1423, 16 had mCSCC and 10 had laCSCC. The median age was 73 years (52 to 88 years); 81% of patients were male; 92% of patients were White; the ECOG PS was 0 (38%) and 1 (62%); 58% of patients had received at least 1 prior anti-cancer systemic therapy; 92% of patients had received prior cancer-related surgery and 81% had received prior radiotherapy. One patient in the mCSCC group was dosed at 1 mg/kg. The rest received 3 mg/kg every 2 weeks. With a median duration of follow-up of 13.3 months, the confirmed ORR was 50% (95% CI: 30, 70); all responses were PRs. The median time to response was 1.9 months (range: 1.7 to 7.3 months) and 85% of responders had a DOR ≥ 6 months.

14.2 Basal Cell Carcinoma (BCC)

The efficacy of LIBTAYO in 112 patients with advanced basal cell carcinoma (BCC) [unresectable locally advanced (laBCC) or metastatic (nodal or distant) (mBCC)] who had progressed on hedgehog pathway inhibitor (HHI) therapy, had not had an objective response after 9 months on HHI therapy, or were intolerant of prior HHI therapy was evaluated in Study 1620 (NCT03132636), an open-label, multi-center, non-randomized study. The study excluded patients with autoimmune disease that required systemic therapy with immunosuppressant agents within 5 years; history of solid organ transplant; prior treatment with anti–PD-1/PD-L1 therapy or other immune check point inhibitor therapy; infection with HIV, hepatitis B or hepatitis C; or ECOG performance score (PS) ≥ 2.

(Figure 47. Basal cell carcinoma of the skin).

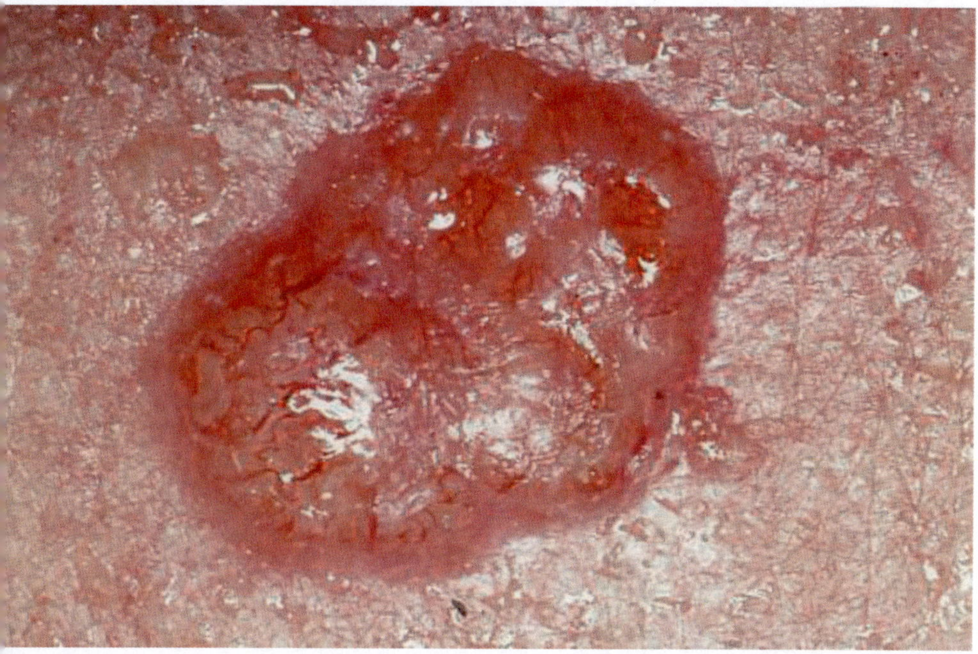

(This image is by No machine-readable author provided. John Hendrix assumed (based on copyright claims). - No machine-readable source provided. Own work assumed (based on copyright claims)., Public Domain, https://commons.wikimedia.org/w/index.php?curid=1216868; en.wikipedia.org/wiki/Basal-cell_carcinoma#/media/File:Basal_cell_carcinoma.jpg. the copyright holder of this work, release this work into the public domain. No changes were made to this image).

Patients received LIBTAYO 350 mg every 3 weeks for up to 93 weeks until disease progression, unacceptable toxicity, or completion of planned treatment. Tumor assessments were performed every 9 weeks for the first 45 weeks of treatment and every 12 weeks thereafter.

(Figure 48. Palisading in nodular basal cell cancer. H&E stain).

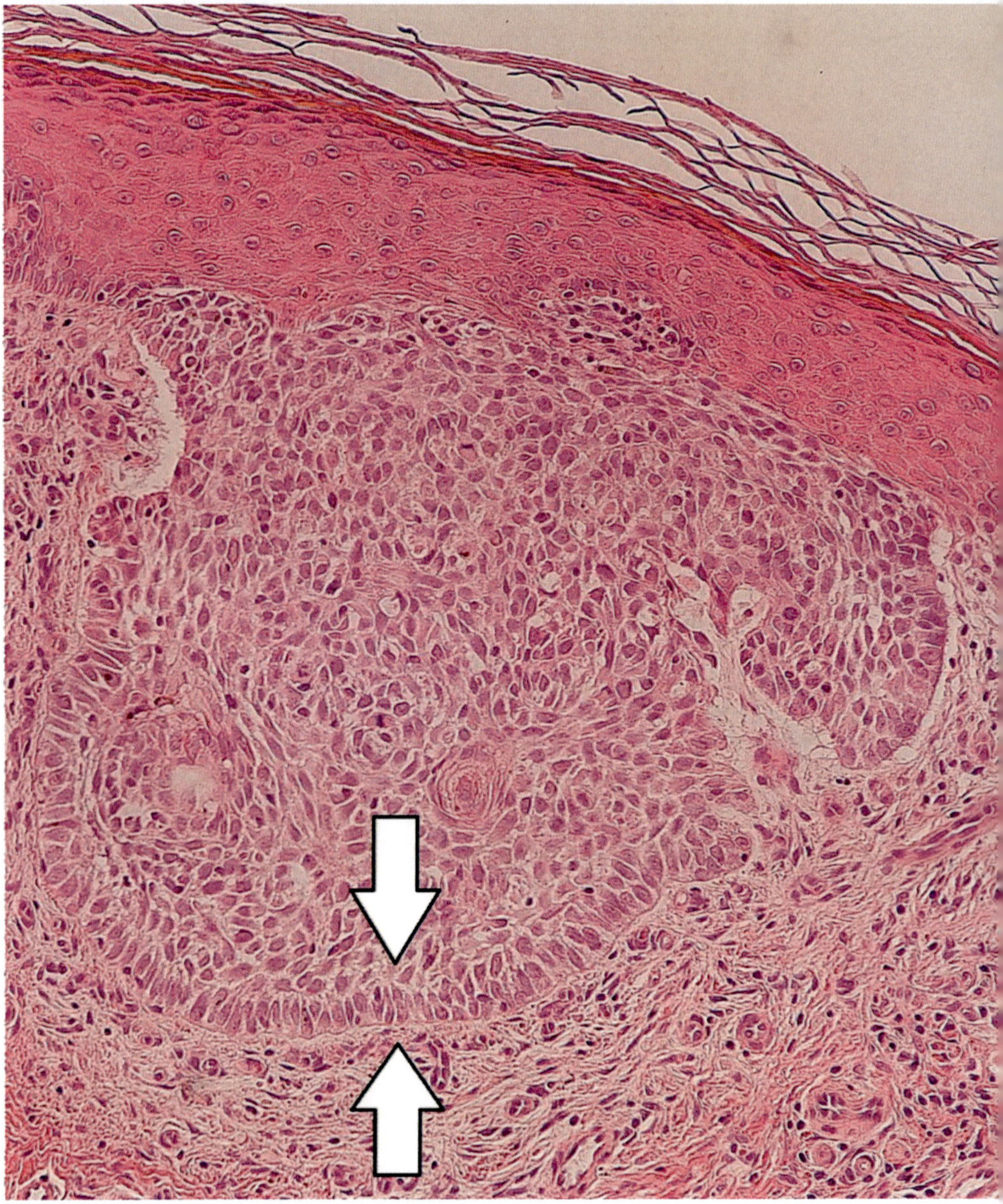

(This image is by Mikael Häggström, M.D. - Own work, CC0, https://commons.wikimedia.org/w/index.php?curid=82523193; /en.wikipedia.org/wiki/Basal-cell_carcinoma#/media/File:Palisading_in_basal_cell_cancer.jpg. This file is made available under the Creative Commons CC0 1.0 Universal Public Domain Dedication. No changes were made to this image).

The major efficacy outcome measures were confirmed objective response rate (ORR) and duration of response (DOR) as assessed by independent central review

(ICR). For patients with mBCC without externally visible target lesions, ORR was determined by Response Evaluation Criteria in Solid Tumors (RECIST 1.1). For patients with externally visible target lesions (laBCC and mBCC), ORR was determined by a composite endpoint that integrated ICR assessments of radiologic data (RECIST 1.1) and digital medical photography (WHO criteria). A total of 112 patients with advanced BCC were included in the efficacy analysis of Study 1620. Of these, 25% had mBCC and 75% had laBCC. In patients with laBCC, the median age was 70 years (42 to 89 years); 67% were male; 68% were White; 61% had ECOG PS 0 and 39% had ECOG PS 1; 83% had received at least 1 prior cancer-related surgery; and 50% had received prior radiotherapy. In patients with mBCC, the median age was 65.5 years (38 to 90 years); 82% were male; 79% were White; 57% had ECOG PS 0 and 43% had ECOG PS 1; 82% had received at least 1 prior cancer-related surgery; and 61% had received prior radiotherapy. Among patients with mBCC, 32% had distant metastases only, 14% had nodal disease only, and 54% had both distant and nodal disease.

For responding patients, the median time to response was 3.2 months (range 2.1 to 10.5 months) for the mBCC group and 4.2 months (range 2.1 to 13.4 months) for the laBCC group. The confirmed objective response rate was 21% in the metastatic BCC group and 29% in the locally advance BCC group. The median duration of response in months was not reached in either group.

Non-Small Cell Lung Cancer (NSCLC)

First-line treatment of NSCLC with LIBTAYO as a single agent

The efficacy of LIBTAYO was evaluated in Study 1624 (NCT03088540), a randomized, multicenter, open-label, active-controlled trial in 710 patients with locally advanced NSCLC who were not candidates for surgical resection or definitive chemoradiation, or with metastatic NSCLC. Only patients whose tumors had high PD-L1 expression [Tumor Proportion Score (TPS) ≥ 50%] as determined by an immunohistochemistry assay using the PD-L1 IHC 22C3 pharmDx kit and who had not received prior systemic treatment for metastatic NSCLC were eligible. Patients with EGFR, ALK or ROS1 genomic tumor aberrations; a medical condition that required systemic immunosuppression; autoimmune disease that required systemic therapy within 2 years of treatment; or who had never smoked were ineligible.

Patients with a history of brain metastases were eligible if they had been adequately treated and had neurologically returned to baseline for at least 2 weeks prior to randomization.

Randomization was stratified by histology (non-squamous vs squamous) and geographic region (Europe vs Asia vs Rest of world). Patients were randomized (1:1) to receive LIBTAYO 350 mg intravenously (IV) every 3 weeks for up to 108 weeks or a platinum-doublet chemotherapy regimen for 4 to 6 cycles followed by optional pemetrexed maintenance for patients with non-squamous histology who received a pemetrexed-containing regimen. Treatment with LIBTAYO continued until RECIST 1.1-defined progressive disease, unacceptable toxicity, or up to 108 weeks. Patients who experienced IRC-assessed RECIST 1.1- defined progressive disease on LIBTAYO therapy were permitted to continue treatment with LIBTAYO (up to an additional 108 weeks) with the addition of 4 cycles of histology-specific chemotherapy until further progression was observed. Of the 203 patients randomized to receive chemotherapy who had IRC-assessed RECIST 1.1-defined disease progression, 150 (74%) patients crossed over to treatment with LIBTAYO. Assessment of tumor status was performed every 9 weeks.

The major efficacy outcome measures were overall survival (OS) and progression-free survival (PFS). An additional efficacy outcome measure was overall response rate (ORR). The study population characteristics were: median age of 63 years (range: 31 to 84), 45% age 65 or older; 85% male; 86% White, 11% Asian; and 0.6% Black. Nine percent were Hispanic or Latino. Twenty-seven percent had ECOG PS 0 and 73% had ECOG PS 1; 84% had metastatic disease and 16% had stage IIIB or IIIC disease and were not candidates for surgical resection or definitive chemoradiation per investigator assessment; 56% had non-squamous and 44% had squamous histology; and 12% had history of treated brain metastases at baseline.

The trial demonstrated a statistically significant improvement in OS and PFS for patients randomized to LIBTAYO as compared with chemotherapy.

5.4. JEMPERLI (dostarlimab) in combination with carboplatin and paclitaxel, followed by JEMPERLI as a single agent, is indicated

- for the treatment of adult patients with **primary advanced or recurrent endometrial cancer (EC).**
- JEMPERLI, as a single agent, is indicated for the treatment of adult patients with **mismatch repair deficient (dMMR) recurrent or advanced EC**, as determined by an FDA-approved test, that has progressed on or following prior treatment with a platinum-containing regimen in any setting and are not candidates for curative surgery or radiation
- JEMPERLI, as a single agent, is indicated for the treatment of adult patients with **dMMR recurrent or advanced solid tumors**, as determined by an FDA-approved test, that have progressed on or following prior treatment and who have no satisfactory alternative treatment options. This indication is approved under accelerated approval based on tumor response rate and durability of response. Continued approval for this indication may be contingent upon verification and description of clinical benefit in a confirmatory trial(s).

12.1 MECHANISM OF ACTION

Binding of the PD-1 ligands, PD-L1 and PD-L2, to the PD-1 receptor found on T cells inhibits T-cell proliferation and cytokine production. Upregulation of PD-1 ligands occurs in some tumors, and signalling through this pathway can contribute to inhibition of active T-cell immune surveillance of tumors. Dostarlimab-gxly is a humanized monoclonal antibody of the IgG4 isotype that binds to the PD-1 receptor and blocks its interaction with PD-L1 and PD-L2, releasing PD-1 pathway-mediated inhibition of the immune response, including the anti-tumor immune response. In syngeneic mouse tumor models, blocking PD-1 activity resulted in decreased tumor growth.

DOSAGE AND ADMINISTRATION

Patient Selection Single Agent

Select patients for treatment with JEMPERLI as a single agent based on the presence of dMMR in tumor specimens in:

- **recurrent or advanced endometrial cancer (EC)**

• **recurrent or advanced solid tumors**. Information on FDA-approved tests for the detection of dMMR status is available at https://www.fda.gov/companiondiagnostics.

Because the effect of prior chemotherapy on test results for dMMR in patients with high-grade gliomas is unclear, it is recommended to test for this marker in the primary tumor specimen obtained prior to initiation of temozolomide chemotherapy in patients with high-grade gliomas.

Recommended Dosage of JEMPERLI

Indication

- Combination Therapy - Adults with primary advanced or recurrent EC Monotherapy

Recommended Dosage Duration/Timing of Treatment

500 mg JEMPERLI every 3 weeks for 6 cycles in combination with carboplatin and paclitaxel followed by 1,000 mg JEMPERLI as monotherapy every 6 weeks for all cycles thereafter. Administer JEMPERLI prior to carboplatin and paclitaxel when given on the same day.

- Adults with dMMR recurrent or advanced EC and dMMR recurrent or advanced solid tumors 500 mg JEMPERLI every 3 weeks for 4 cycles followed by 1,000 mg JEMPERLI every 6 weeks for all cycles thereafter. until disease progression, unacceptable toxicity, or up to 3 years, disease progression or unacceptable toxicity.

Dosage Modifications for Adverse Reactions

- No dose reductions of JEMPERLI are recommended. In general, withhold JEMPERLI for severe (Grade 3) immune-mediated adverse reactions. Permanently discontinue JEMPERLI for life-threatening (Grade 4) immune-mediated adverse reactions, recurrent severe (Grade 3) immune-mediated reactions that require systemic immunosuppressive treatment, or an inability to reduce corticosteroid dose to 10 mg or less of prednisone equivalent per day within 12 weeks of initiating steroids. Dosage modifications for JEMPERLI for adverse reactions that require management different from these general guidelines are summarized in Table 2.

Adverse Reaction	Severity[a]	Dosage Modification
Pneumonitis	Grade 2 Grade 3 or 4 or recurrent Grade 2	Withhold[b] Permanently discontinue
Colitis	Grade 2 or 3 Grade 4	Withhold[b] Permanently discontinue
Hepatitis with no tumor involvement of the liver	AST or ALT increases to more than 3 and up to 8 times ULN or Total bilirubin increases to more than 1.5 and up to 3 times ULN	Withhold[b]
Hepatitis with no tumor involvement of the liver	AST or ALT increases to more than 8 times ULN or Total bilirubin increases to more than 3 times ULN	Permanently discontinue
Hepatitis with tumor involvement of the liver[c]	Baseline AST or ALT is more than 1 and up to 3 times ULN and increases to more than 5 and up to 10 times ULN or Baseline AST or ALT is more than 3 and up to 5 times ULN and increases to more than 8 and up to 10 times ULN	Withhold[b]
	AST or ALT increases to more than 10 times ULN or Total bilirubin	Permanently discontinue

	increases to more than 3 times ULN	
Endocrinopathies	Grade 2, 3, or 4	Withhold until clinically stable or permanently discontinue, depending on severity[b]
Nephritis with renal dysfunction	Grade 2 or 3 increased blood creatinine	Withhold[b]
	Grade 4 increased blood creatinine	Permanently discontinue
Exfoliative dermatologic conditions	Suspected SJS, TEN, or DRESS	Withhold[b]
	Confirmed SJS, TEN, or DRESS	Permanently discontinue
Myocarditis	Grade 2, 3, or 4	Permanently discontinue
Neurological toxicities	Grade 2	Withhold[b]
	Grade 3 or 4	Permanently discontinue
Other adverse reactions		
Infusion-related reactions	Grade 1 or 2	Interrupt or slow the rate of infusion
	Grade 3 or 4	Permanently discontinue

AST = aspartate aminotransferase, ALT = alanine aminotransferase, ULN = upper limit of normal, SJS = Stevens-Johnson syndrome, TEN = toxic epidermal necrolysis, DRESS = drug rash with eosinophilia and systemic symptoms. [a] Based on National Cancer Institute Common Terminology Criteria for Adverse Events, Version 4.0. [b] Resume in patients with complete or partial resolution (Grade 0 to 1) after corticosteroid taper. Permanently discontinue if no complete or partial resolution within 12 weeks of initiating steroids or inability to reduce prednisone to less than 10 mg/day (or equivalent) within 12 weeks of initiating steroids. [c] If AST and ALT are less than or equal to ULN at baseline in patients with liver involvement, withhold or permanently discontinue JEMPERLI based on recommendations for hepatitis with no liver involvement.

Preparation and Administration Preparation for Intravenous Infusion

- Visually inspect the solution for particulate matter and discoloration. The solution is clear to slightly opalescent, colorless to yellow. Discard the vial if visible particles are observed.
- Do not shake.
- JEMPERLI is compatible with an infusion bag made of polyolefin, ethylene vinyl acetate, or polyvinyl chloride with di(2-ethylhexyl) phthalate (DEHP).
- For the 500-mg dose, withdraw 10 mL of JEMPERLI from a vial using a disposable sterile syringe made of polypropylene and dilute into an intravenous infusion bag containing 0.9% Sodium Chloride Injection, USP or 5% Dextrose Injection, USP to a final concentration between 2 to 10 mg/mL (maximum 250 mL).
- For the 1,000-mg dose, withdraw 10 mL from each of 2 vials (withdraw 20 mL total) and dilute into an intravenous bag containing 0.9% Sodium Chloride Injection, USP or 5% Dextrose Injection, USP to a final concentration between 4 to 10 mg/mL (maximum 250 mL).
- Mix diluted solution by gentle inversion. Do not shake.
- Discard any unused portion left in the vial.

Storage of Infusion Solution Store in the original carton until time of preparation in order to protect from light.

The prepared dose may be stored either

- At room temperature for no more than 6 hours from the time of preparation until the end of infusion.

• Under refrigeration at 2°C to 8°C (36ºF to 46ºF) for no more than 24 hours from time of preparation until end of infusion. If refrigerated, allow the diluted solution to come to room temperature prior to administration. Discard after 6 hours at room temperature or after 24 hours under refrigeration. Do not freeze.

Administration

Administer infusion solution intravenously over 30 minutes through an intravenous line using tubing made of polyvinyl chloride or platinum cured silicon; fittings made of polyvinyl chloride or polycarbonate; and a sterile, non-pyrogenic, low-protein binding, 0.2-micron, in-line or add-on filter.

JEMPERLI must not be administered as an intravenous push or bolus injection. Do not co-administer other drugs through the same infusion line.

DOSAGE FORMS AND STRENGTHS

Injection: 500 mg/10 mL (50 mg/mL) clear to slightly opalescent, colorless to yellow solution in a single-dose vial for intravenous infusion after dilution.

CONTRAINDICATIONS

None

WARNINGS AND PRECAUTIONS

Severe and Fatal Immune-Mediated Adverse Reactions

JEMPERLI is a monoclonal antibody that belongs to a class of drugs that bind to either the programmed death receptor-1 (PD-1) or PD-ligand 1 (PD-L1), blocking the PD-1/PD-L1 pathway, thereby removing inhibition of the immune response, potentially breaking peripheral tolerance, and inducing immune-mediated adverse reactions.

Important immune-mediated adverse reactions listed in WARNINGS AND PRECAUTIONS may not include all possible severe and fatal immune-mediated reactions. Immune-mediated adverse reactions, which can be severe or fatal, can occur in any organ system or tissue. Immune-mediated adverse reactions can occur at any time after starting a PD-1/PD-L1–blocking antibody. While immune-mediated adverse reactions usually manifest during treatment with PD-1/PD-L1–blocking antibodies, they can also manifest after discontinuation of PD-1/PD-L1–blocking antibodies. Early identification and management of immune-mediated adverse reactions are essential to ensure safe use of PD-1/PD-L1–blocking antibodies. Monitor closely for symptoms and signs that may be clinical manifestations of underlying immune-mediated adverse reactions. Evaluate liver enzymes, creatinine, and thyroid function tests at baseline and periodically during treatment. In cases of suspected immune-mediated adverse reactions, initiate appropriate workup to exclude alternative etiologies, including infection. Institute medical management promptly, including specialty consultation as appropriate.

Withhold or permanently discontinue JEMPERLI depending on severity

In general, if JEMPERLI requires interruption or discontinuation, administer systemic corticosteroids (1 to 2 mg/kg/day prednisone or equivalent) until improvement to Grade 1 or less. Upon improvement to Grade 1 or less, initiate corticosteroid taper and continue to taper over at least 1 month. Consider administration of other systemic immunosuppressants in patients whose immune-mediated adverse reaction is not controlled with corticosteroids. Toxicity management guidelines for adverse reactions that do not necessarily require systemic steroids (e.g., endocrinopathies, dermatologic reactions) are discussed below.

Immune-Mediated Pneumonitis

JEMPERLI can cause immune-mediated pneumonitis, which can be fatal. In patients treated with other PD-1/PD-L1–blocking antibodies, the incidence of pneumonitis is higher in patients who have received prior thoracic radiation. Immune-mediated pneumonitis occurred in 2.3% (14/605) of patients receiving JEMPERLI, including Grade 2 (1.3%), Grade 3 (0.8%) and Grade 4 (0.2%) pneumonitis. Pneumonitis led to discontinuation of JEMPERLI in 1.3% of patients. Systemic corticosteroids were required in 79% (11/14) of patients with pneumonitis. Pneumonitis resolved in 11 of the 14 patients. JEMPERLI was withheld for 9 patients. Five patients reinitiated JEMPERLI after symptom improvement; of these, 2 patients had recurrence of pneumonitis.

Immune-Mediated Colitis

JEMPERLI can cause immune-mediated colitis. **Cytomegalovirus infection/reactivation** have occurred in patients with corticosteroid-refractory immune-mediated colitis treated with PD-1/PD-L1–blocking antibodies. In cases of corticosteroid-refractory colitis, consider repeating infectious workup to exclude alternative etiologies. Immune-mediated colitis occurred in 1.3% (8/605) of patients receiving JEMPERLI, including Grade 2 (0.7%) and Grade 3 (0.7%) adverse reactions. Colitis led to discontinuation of JEMPERLI in 1 (0.2%) patient. Systemic corticosteroids were required in 75% (6/8) of patients with colitis. Colitis resolved in 5 of the 8 patients. Of the 4 patients in whom JEMPERLI was withheld for colitis, all reinitiated treatment with JEMPERLI; of these, 1 patient had recurrence of colitis.

(Figure 49. A lung pneumocyte infected by human cytomegalovirus. The central cell displays the dramatically enlarged nuclei characteristic of CMV. Histopathology of lung shows cytomegalic pneumocyte containing characteristic intranuclear inclusions).

(This image is Transferred from en.wikipedia to Commons.This media comes from the Centers for Disease Control and Prevention's Public Health Image Library (PHIL), with identification number #958, Public Domain, Image credit: CDC/Dr. Edwin P. Ewing, Jr. (PHIL #958), 1982.https://commons.wikimedia.org/w/index.php?curid=1880647; en.wikipedia.org/wiki/Cytomegalovirus#/media/File:Cytomegalovirus_01.jpg. This image is a work of the Centers for Disease Control and Prevention, part of the United States Department of Health and Human Services, taken or made as part of an employee's official duties. As a work of the U.S. federal government, the image is in the public domain. No changes were made to this image).

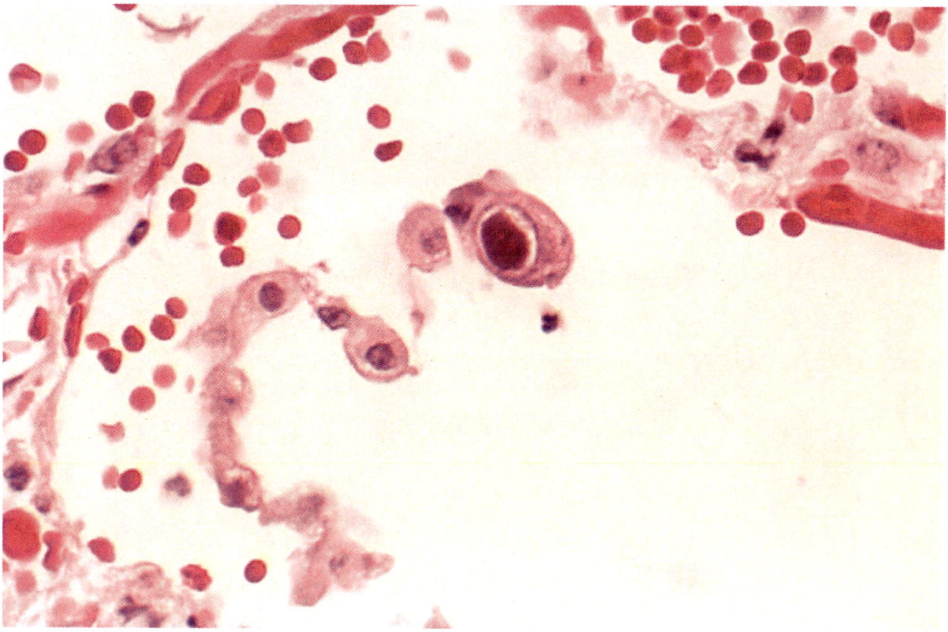

Immune-Mediated Hepatitis

JEMPERLI can cause immune-mediated hepatitis, which can be fatal. Immune-mediated hepatitis occurred in 0.5% (3/605) of patients receiving JEMPERLI, all were Grade 3. Hepatitis led to discontinuation of JEMPERLI in 1 (0.2%) patient. Systemic corticosteroids were required in 2 patients with hepatitis and the events resolved in 2 of the 3 patients.

Immune-Mediated Endocrinopathies

Adrenal Insufficiency

JEMPERLI can cause primary or secondary adrenal insufficiency. For Grade 2 or higher adrenal insufficiency, initiate symptomatic treatment per institutional guidelines, including hormone replacement as clinically indicated. Withhold or permanently discontinue JEMPERLI depending on severity. Adrenal insufficiency occurred in 1.2% (7/605) patients receiving JEMPERLI, including Grade 2 (0.5%) and Grade 3 (0.7%). Adrenal insufficiency resulted in discontinuation in 1 (0.2%) patient and resolved in 4 of the 7 patients. Of the 4 patients in whom JEMPERLI was withheld for adrenal insufficiency, all reinitiated treatment with JEMPERLI. Systemic corticosteroids were required in 5 of the 7 patients with adrenal insufficiency.

Hypophysitis

JEMPERLI can cause immune-mediated hypophysitis. Hypophysitis can present with acute symptoms associated with mass effect such as headache, photophobia, or visual field cuts. Hypophysitis can cause hypopituitarism. Initiate hormone replacement as clinically indicated. Withhold or permanently discontinue JEMPERLI depending on severity

JEMPERLI in Combination with Carboplatin and Paclitaxel

Hypophysitis (Grade 3) occurred in 0.4% (1/241) of patients receiving JEMPERLI in combination with carboplatin and paclitaxel. Systemic corticosteroids were required, and the event resolved. JEMPERLI was withheld and the patient reinitiated treatment.

JEMPERLI as a Single Agent

Hypophysitis (Grade 2) occurred in 0.2% (1/605) of patients receiving JEMPERLI as a single agent. Systemic corticosteroids were required, and the event did not resolve. JEMPERLI was withheld and the patient reinitiated treatment.

Thyroid Disorders

JEMPERLI can cause immune-mediated thyroid disorders. Thyroiditis can present with or without endocrinopathy. Hypothyroidism can follow hyperthyroidism. Initiate thyroid hormone replacement or medical management of hyperthyroidism as clinically indicated. Withhold or permanently discontinue JEMPERLI depending on severity

Thyroiditis

Thyroiditis occurred in 0.5% (3/605) of patients receiving JEMPERLI; all were Grade 2. Systemic corticosteroids were required in 1 of 3 patients and anti-thyroid therapy was required for 2 of 3 patients with thyroiditis. JEMPERLI was withheld for 1 patient and the patient reinitiated treatment. None of the events of thyroiditis resolved; there were no discontinuations of JEMPERLI due to thyroiditis.

Hypothyroidism

JEMPERLI in Combination with Carboplatin and Paclitaxel

Hypothyroidism occurred in 12% (30/241) of patients receiving JEMPERLI in combination with carboplatin and paclitaxel, all of which were Grade 2. Hypothyroidism led to discontinuation of JEMPERLI in 1 patient and resolved in 23% (7/30) of patients. JEMPERLI was withheld for 5 patients and all reinitiated treatment with JEMPERLI. Thyroid hormone replacement was required for 27 of the 30 patients with hypothyroidism.

JEMPERLI as a Single Agent

Hypothyroidism occurred in 8% (46/605) of patients receiving JEMPERLI as a single agent, all of which were Grade 2. Hypothyroidism did not lead to discontinuation of JEMPERLI and resolved in 37% (17/46) of patients. JEMPERLI was withheld for 2 patients and both reinitiated treatment. Thyroid hormone replacement therapy was required for 45 of the 46 patients with hypothyroidism.

JEMPERLI in Combination with Carboplatin and Paclitaxel

Hyperthyroidism occurred in 3.3% (8/241) of patients receiving JEMPERLI in combination with carboplatin and paclitaxel, including Grade 2 (2.9%) and Grade 3 (0.4%). Hyperthyroidism did not lead to discontinuation of JEMPERLI and resolved in 75% (6/8) of patients. JEMPERLI was withheld for 1 patient and the patient reinitiated treatment. Anti-thyroid therapy was required for 2 of the 8 patients while systemic corticosteroids were required for 1 of the 8 patients with hyperthyroidism.

JEMPERLI as a Single Agent

Hyperthyroidism occurred in 2.3% (14/605) of patients receiving JEMPERLI as a single agent, including Grade 2 (2.1%) and Grade 3 (0.2%). Hyperthyroidism did not lead to discontinuation of JEMPERLI and resolved in 71% (10/14) of the 14 patients. JEMPERLI was withheld for 2 patients and both reinitiated treatment. Anti-thyroid therapy was required for 10 of the 14 patients with hyperthyroidism.

Type 1 Diabetes Mellitus Which Can Present with Diabetic Ketoacidosis

JEMPERLI can cause type 1 diabetes mellitus, which can present with diabetic ketoacidosis. Monitor patients for hyperglycemia or other signs and symptoms of diabetes. Initiate treatment with insulin as clinically indicated. Withhold or permanently discontinue JEMPERLI depending on severity

JEMPERLI in Combination with Carboplatin and Paclitaxel

Type 1 diabetes mellitus (Grade 3) occurred in 0.4% (1/241) of patients receiving JEMPERLI in combination with carboplatin and paclitaxel. Type 1 diabetes mellitus led to withholding JEMPERLI; the patient reinitiated treatment and required long-term insulin therapy.

JEMPERLI as a Single Agent

Type 1 diabetes mellitus occurred in 0.2% (1/605) of patients receiving JEMPERLI as a single agent, which was Grade 3. Type 1 diabetes mellitus did not result in treatment discontinuation and did not resolve.

Immune-Mediated Nephritis with Renal Dysfunction

JEMPERLI can cause immune-mediated nephritis, which can be fatal. Nephritis, including tubulointerstitial nephritis, occurred in 0.5% (3/605) of patients receiving JEMPERLI; all were Grade 2. Nephritis led to discontinuation of JEMPERLI in 1 (0.2%) patient and resolved in all patients. JEMPERLI was withheld for 1 patient and the patient reinitiated treatment. Systemic corticosteroids were required in 2 of the 3 patients experiencing nephritis.

(Further clinical information on these immune-mediated disorders is given in the section on nivolumab)

Immune-Mediated Dermatologic Adverse Reactions

JEMPERLI can cause immune-mediated rash or dermatitis. Bullous and exfoliative dermatitis, including Stevens-Johnson syndrome (SJS), toxic epidermal necrolysis (TEN), and drug rash with eosinophilia and systemic symptoms (DRESS), have occurred with PD-1/PD-L1–blocking antibodies. Topical emollients and/or topical corticosteroids may be adequate to treat mild to moderate non-bullous/exfoliative rashes. Withhold or permanently discontinue JEMPERLI depending on severity

Other Immune-Mediated Adverse Reactions

The following clinically significant immune-mediated adverse reactions occurred in <1% of the 605 patients treated with JEMPERLI or were reported with the use of other PD-1/PD-L1– blocking antibodies. Severe or fatal cases have been reported for some of these adverse reactions.

Nervous System

Meningitis, encephalitis, myelitis and demyelination, myasthenic syndrome/myasthenia gravis, Guillain-Barré syndrome, nerve paresis, autoimmune neuropathy.

Cardiac/Vascular

Myocarditis, pericarditis, vasculitis.

Ocular

Uveitis, iritis, other ocular inflammatory toxicities. Some cases can be associated with retinal detachment. Various grades of visual impairment to include blindness can occur. If uveitis occurs in combination with other immune-mediated adverse reactions, consider a **Vogt-Koyanagi-Harada–like syndrome**, as this may require treatment with systemic steroids to reduce the risk of permanent vision loss.

(*Figure 50. Vogt-Koyanagi-Harada–like syndrome showing uveitis with poliosis of the eyelashes*)

(This image is by National Eye Institute - [1], Public Domain, https://commons.wikimedia.org/w/index.php?curid=4203573; https://en.wikipedia.org/wiki/Vogt%E2%80%93Koyanagi%E2%80%93Harada_disease#/media/File:Poliosis_VKHS.JPG. This work is in the public domain in the United States because it is a work prepared by an officer or employee of the United States Government as part of that person's official duties under the terms of Title 17, Chapter 1, Section 105 of the US Code. No changes were made to this image).

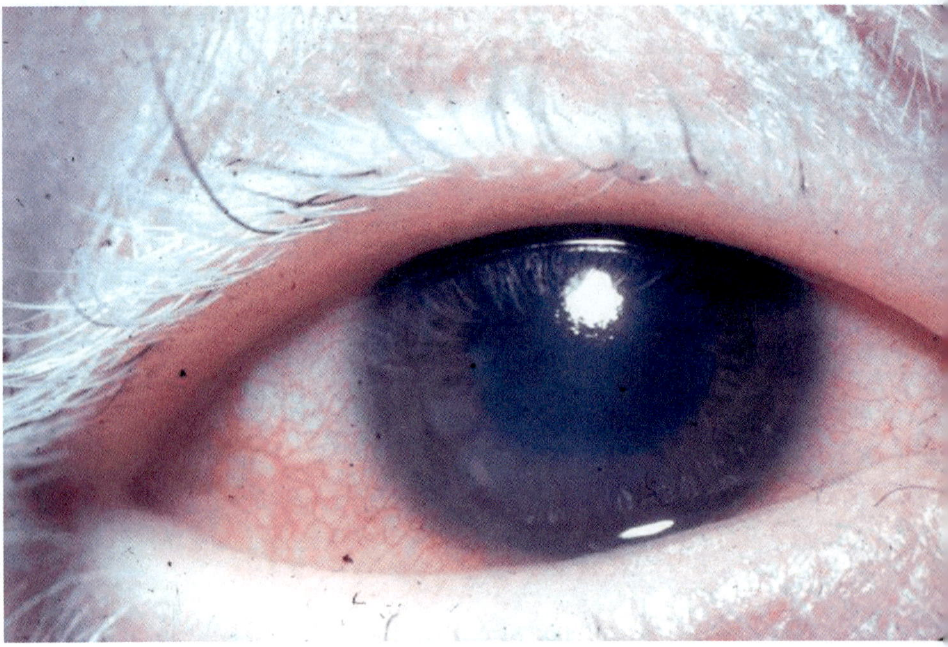

Gastrointestinal

Pancreatitis, including increases in serum amylase and lipase levels, gastritis, duodenitis.

Musculoskeletal and Connective Tissue

Myositis/polymyositis, rhabdomyolysis and associated sequelae including renal failure, arthritis, polymyalgia rheumatica.

Endocrine

Hypoparathyroidism.

Other (Hematologic/Immune)

Autoimmune hemolytic anemia, aplastic anemia, hemophagocytic lymphohistiocytosis, systemic inflammatory response syndrome, histiocytic necrotizing lymphadenitis (Kikuchi lymphadenitis), sarcoidosis, immune thrombocytopenia, solid organ transplant rejection.

Infusion-Related Reactions

Severe or life-threatening infusion-related reactions have been reported with PD-1/PD-L1– blocking antibodies. Severe infusion-related reactions (Grade 3) occurred in 0.2% (1/605) of patients receiving JEMPERLI. All patients recovered from the infusion-related reactions. Monitor patients for signs and symptoms of infusion-related reactions. Interrupt or slow the rate of infusion or permanently discontinue JEMPERLI based on severity of reaction

Complications of allogeneic hematopoietic stem cell transplantation (HSCT)

Fatal and other serious complications can occur in patients who receive an allogeneic hematopoietic stem cell transplantation (HSCT) before or after being treated with a PD-1/PD-L1–blocking antibody. Transplant-related complications include hyperacute graft-versus-host disease (GVHD), acute GVHD, chronic GVHD, hepatic veno-occlusive disease after reduced intensity conditioning, and steroid-requiring febrile syndrome (without an identified infectious cause). These complications may occur despite intervening therapy between PD-1/PD-L1 blockade and allogeneic HSCT. Follow patients closely for evidence of transplant-related complications and intervene promptly. Consider the benefit versus risks of treatment with a PD-1/PD-L1–blocking antibody prior to or after an allogeneic HSCT.

The following clinically significant immune-mediated adverse reactions occurred in 1 year and 19% were exposed for >2 years.

Primary Advanced or Recurrent Endometrial Cancer:

JEMPERLI in Combination with Carboplatin and Paclitaxel The safety of JEMPERLI in patients with primary advanced or recurrent EC was evaluated in RUBY. Patients received JEMPERLI 500 mg (n = 241) or placebo (n = 246) in combination with carboplatin and paclitaxel every 3 weeks for 6 cycles followed by JEMPERLI 1,000 mg or placebo every 6 weeks until disease progression or unacceptable toxicity. Among the 241 patients, 38.6% were exposed for >1 year and 24.1% were exposed for >2 years. Serious adverse reactions occurred in 39% of patients receiving JEMPERLI in combination with carboplatin and paclitaxel; the most common serious adverse reactions were sepsis, including urosepsis (3.7%), and pulmonary embolism (3.3%). Fatal adverse reactions occurred in 1.2% of patients receiving JEMPERLI including septic shock (0.8%) and myelosuppression (0.4%). In patients receiving JEMPERLI in combination with carboplatin and paclitaxel, JEMPERLI was permanently discontinued due to adverse reactions in 46 patients (19%). Adverse reactions that required permanent discontinuation in ≥2 patients included 3 cases (1.2%) of maculo-papular rash, and 2 cases (0.8%) each of increased alanine aminotransferase (ALT), increased aspartate aminotransferase (AST), diarrhea, pancreatitis, fatigue, pneumonitis, and arthralgia. Dosage interruptions due to an adverse reaction occurred in 37% of patients who received JEMPERLI in combination with carboplatin and paclitaxel.

Adverse reactions that required dosage interruption in ≥5% of patients who received JEMPERLI in combination with carboplatin and paclitaxel were anemia, thrombocytopenia, and peripheral neuropathy.

The most common adverse reactions, including laboratory abnormalities (≥20%), were decreased hemoglobin, increased creatinine, peripheral neuropathy, decreased white blood cell count, fatigue, nausea, alopecia, decreased platelets, increased glucose, decreased lymphocytes, decreased magnesium, decreased neutrophils, increased AST, arthralgia, rash, constipation, diarrhea, increased ALT, decreased potassium, decreased albumin, decreased sodium, increased alkaline phosphatase, abdominal pain, dyspnea, decreased appetite, increased amylase, decreased phosphate, urinary tract infection, and vomiting. A fatal adverse reaction occurred in one patient (0.7%) who received JEMPERLI, due to concurrent immune-mediated encephalitis and urinary tract infection. Serious adverse reactions occurred in 38% of patients receiving JEMPERLI. Serious adverse reactions in >2% of patients included urinary tract infection (4%), sepsis (3.3%), acute kidney injury (2.7%), and abdominal pain (2.7%).

JEMPERLI was permanently discontinued due to adverse reactions in 15 (10%) patients, including increased transaminases, sepsis, bronchitis, pneumonitis, rash, pruritus, pancreatitis, encephalitis, and nephritis.

Dosage interruptions due to an adverse reaction occurred in 28% of patients who received JEMPERLI. Adverse reactions that required dosage interruption in >1% of patients who received JEMPERLI were anemia, diarrhea, asthenia, colitis, sepsis, and pneumonitis.

The most common adverse reactions (≥20%) were fatigue/asthenia, anemia, nausea, diarrhea, constipation, vomiting, and rash.

14. CLINICAL STUDIES

No other check point inhibitors have yet received FDA approval for advanced solid tumors without any other satisfactory alternative treatment. Therefore, this section on JEMPERLI will focus on that subject

14.2 Mismatch Repair Deficient Recurrent or Advanced Solid Tumors

The efficacy of JEMPERLI as a single agent was evaluated in GARNET (NCT02715284), a non-randomized, multicenter, open-label, multicohort trial. The efficacy population consisted of a cohort of 209 patients with dMMR recurrent or advanced solid tumors who progressed following systemic therapy and had no satisfactory alternative treatment options.

(Tumor types included in this trial were endometrial carcinoma, colo-rectal carcinoma, small intestinal cancer, gastric cancer, pancreatic carcinoma, biliary tract, neoplasm, liver cancer, ovarian cancer, adrenocortical cancer, breast cancer, esophageal cancer, genital neoplasm, malignant pleural neoplasm, renal cell carcinoma and cancer of unknown origin).

(Figure 51. Cross-section of a human liver at autopsy, showing many large pale tumor deposits which are metastases from pancreatic cancer.

This image is by Haymanj - Self-photographed, Public Domain, https://commons.wikimedia.org/w/index.php?curid=3662694; https://en.wikipedia.org/wiki/Pancreatic_cancer#/media/File:Secondary_tumor_deposits_in_the_liver_from_a_primary_cancer_of_the_pancreas.jpg. The copyright holder of this work has released this work into the public domain. No changes were made to this image).

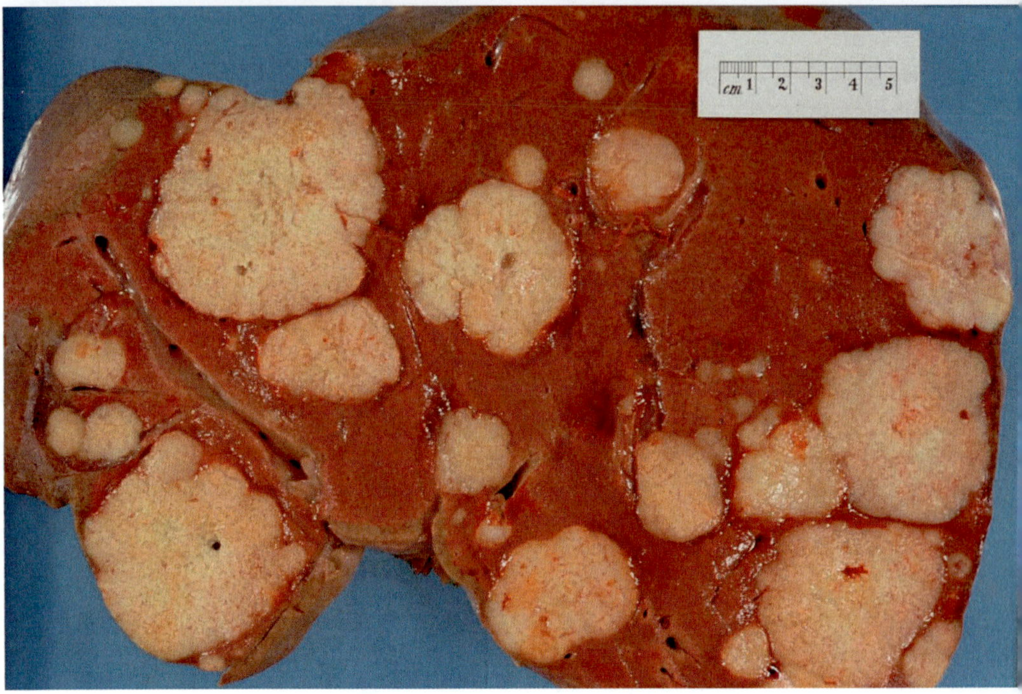

(Figure 52. Gross view of a large adrenocortical carcinoma).

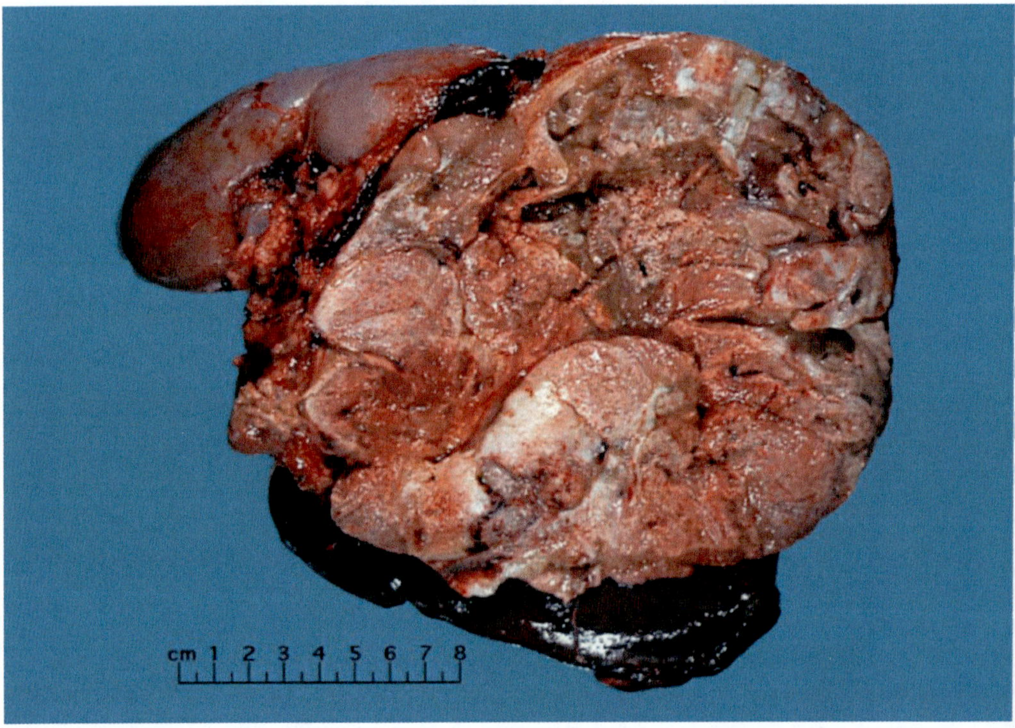

(This image is by AFIP Atlas of Tumor Pathology - [1], Public Domain, https://commons.wikimedia.org/w/index.php?curid=6719487; https://en.wikipedia.org/wiki/Adrenocortical_carcinoma#/media/File:Adrenal_cortical_carcinoma.JPG. This work is in the public domain in the United States because it is a work prepared by an officer or employee of the United States Government as part of that person's official duties under the terms of Title 17, Chapter 1, Section 105 of the US Code. No changes were made to this image).

Patients with dMMR EC must have progressed on or after treatment with a platinum-containing regimen. Patients with dMMR colorectal cancer must have progressed after or been intolerant to a fluoropyrimidine, oxaliplatin, and irinotecan. Patients with prior treatment with PD-1/PD-L1–blocking antibodies or other immune check point inhibitor therapy and patients with autoimmune disease that required systemic therapy with immunosuppressant agents within 2 years were excluded from the trial.

Patients received JEMPERLI 500 mg intravenously every 3 weeks for 4 doses followed by 1,000 mg intravenously every 6 weeks. Treatment continued until disease progression or unacceptable toxicity. The major efficacy outcome measures were ORR and DOR as determined by a BICR according to RECIST v 1.1. The baseline characteristics were female (77%); median age 63 years (47% aged 65 years or older); 63% White, 3% Asian, 2% Black; and Eastern Cooperative Oncology Group Performance Status 0 (39%) or 1 (61%). At time of trial entry, 97.2% of patients (103/106) with non-endometrial dMMR solid tumors had Stage IV disease, and 68.0% (70/103) of patients with dMMR endometrial tumors had FIGO Stage IV disease. Approximately 43% of patients had received 1 prior line of systemic anticancer treatment, 36% had received 2 prior lines, and 21% had received 3 or more prior lines. The dMMR tumor status was retrospectively confirmed using the VENTANA MMR RxDx Panel assay.

The overall response rate was 41%. The complete response rate was 9.1% and the partial response rate was 32.5%. The median duration of response was 34.7 months (range 2.6 to 35.8+ months).

6. PDL-1 INHIBITORS

6.1. TEZOLIMUMAB

TECENTRIQ® (atezolizumab) injection, for intravenous use Initial U.S. Approval: 2016

TECENTRIQ is a programmed death-ligand 1 (PD-L1) blocking antibody indicated:

Urothelial Carcinoma

• for the treatment of adult patients with locally advanced or metastatic urothelial carcinoma who:

o are not eligible for cisplatin-containing chemotherapy and whose tumors express PD-L1 (PD-L1 stained tumor-infiltrating immune cells [IC] covering ≥ 5% of the tumor area), as determined by an FDA-approved test, or

o are not eligible for any platinum-containing chemotherapy regardless of PD-L1 status This indication is approved under accelerated approval based on tumor response rate and duration of response. Continued approval for this indication may be contingent upon verification and description of clinical benefit in a confirmatory trial(s).

Non-Small Cell Lung Cancer (NSCLC)

• as adjuvant treatment following resection and platinum-based chemotherapy for adult patients with Stage II to IIIA NSCLC whose tumors have PD-L1 expression on ≥ 1% of tumor cells, as determined by an FDA-approved test.

• for the first-line treatment of adult patients with metastatic NSCLC whose tumors have high PD-L1 expression (PD-L1 stained ≥ 50% of tumor cells [TC ≥ 50%] or PD-L1 stained tumor-infiltrating immune cells [IC] covering ≥ 10% of the tumor area [IC ≥ 10%]), as determined by an FDAapproved test, with no EGFR or ALK genomic tumor aberrations.

• in combination with bevacizumab, paclitaxel, and carboplatin, for the firstline treatment of adult patients with metastatic non-squamous NSCLC with no EGFR or ALK genomic tumor aberrations.

• in combination with paclitaxel protein-bound and carboplatin for the firstline treatment of adult patients with metastatic non-squamous NSCLC with no EGFR or ALK genomic tumor aberrations

• for the treatment of adult patients with metastatic NSCLC who have disease progression during or following platinum-containing chemotherapy. Patients with EGFR or ALK genomic tumor aberrations should have disease progression on FDA-approved therapy for NSCLC harboring these aberrations prior to receiving TECENTRIQ.

Small Cell Lung Cancer (SCLC)

- in combination with carboplatin and etoposide, for the first-line treatment of adult patients with extensive-stage small cell lung cancer (ES-SCLC).

Hepatocellular Carcinoma (HCC)

- in combination with bevacizumab for the treatment of patients with unresectable or metastatic HCC who have not received prior systemic therapy.

Melanoma

- in combination with cobimetinib and vemurafenib for the treatment of patients with BRAF V600 mutation-positive unresectable or metastatic melanoma

(Unlike current indications for nivolumab, pembrolizumab and cemiplimab, atezolimumab is FDA-approved for the treatment of small cell lung cancer, in addition to other malignacies).

DOSAGE AND ADMINISTRATION

Administer TECENTRIQ intravenously over 60 minutes. If the first infusion is tolerated, all subsequent infusions may be delivered over 30 minutes.

Urothelial Carcinoma

- Administer TECENTRIQ as a single agent as 840 mg every 2 weeks, 1200 mg every 3 weeks, or 1680 mg every 4 weeks.

Non-Small Cell Lung Cancer (NSCLC)

- In the adjuvant setting, administer TECENTRIQ following resection and up to 4 cycles of platinum-based chemotherapy as 840 mg every 2 weeks, 1200 mg every 3 weeks or 1680 mg every 4 weeks for up to 1 year.
- In the metastatic setting, administer TECENTRIQ as 840 mg every 2 weeks, 1200 mg every 3 weeks, or 1680 mg every 4 weeks.

• When administering with chemotherapy with or without bevacizumab, administer TECENTRIQ prior to chemotherapy and bevacizumab when given on the same day.

Small Cell Lung Cancer

• Administer TECENTRIQ as 840 mg every 2 weeks, 1200 mg every 3 weeks, or 1680 mg every 4 weeks. When administering with carboplatin and etoposide, administer TECENTRIQ prior to chemotherapy when given on the same day.

Hepatocellular Carcinoma

• Administer TECENTRIQ as 840 mg every 2 weeks, 1200 mg every 3 weeks, or 1680 mg every 4 weeks. Administer TECENTRIQ prior to bevacizumab when given on the same day. Bevacizumab is administered at 15 mg/kg every 3 weeks.

Melanoma

• Following completion of a 28 day cycle of cobimetinib and vemurafenib, administer TECENTRIQ 840 mg every 2 weeks, 1200 mg every 3 weeks, or 1680 mg every 4 weeks with cobimetinib 60 mg orally once daily (21 days on /7 days off) and vemurafenib 720 mg orally twice daily.

DOSAGE FORMS AND STRENGTHS

Injection: 840 mg/14 mL (60 mg/mL) and 1200 mg/20 mL (60 mg/mL) solution in a single-dose vial.

CONTRAINDICATIONS

None

TECENTRIQ is a programmed death-ligand 1 (PD-L1) blocking antibody indicated:

Urothelial Carcinoma

• for the treatment of adult patients with locally advanced or metastatic urothelial carcinoma who:

o are not eligible for cisplatin-containing chemotherapy and whose tumors express PD-L1 (PD-L1 stained tumor-infiltrating immune cells [IC] covering ≥ 5% of the tumor area), as determined by an FDA-approved test, or

o are not eligible for any platinum-containing chemotherapy regardless of PD-L1 status This indication is approved under accelerated approval based on tumor response rate and duration of response. Continued approval for this indication may be contingent upon verification and description of clinical benefit in a confirmatory trial(s).

Non-Small Cell Lung Cancer (NSCLC)

• as adjuvant treatment following resection and platinum-based chemotherapy for adult patients with Stage II to IIIA NSCLC whose tumors have PD-L1 expression on ≥ 1% of tumor cells, as determined by an FDA-approved test.

• for the first-line treatment of adult patients with metastatic NSCLC whose tumors have high PD-L1 expression (PD-L1 stained ≥ 50% of tumor cells [TC ≥ 50%] or PD-L1 stained tumor-infiltrating immune cells [IC] covering ≥ 10% of the tumor area [IC ≥ 10%]), as determined by an FDA-approved test, with no EGFR or ALK genomic tumor aberrations.

• in combination with bevacizumab, paclitaxel, and carboplatin, for the firstline treatment of adult patients with metastatic non-squamous NSCLC with no EGFR or ALK genomic tumor aberrations.

• in combination with paclitaxel protein-bound and carboplatin for the first line treatment of adult patients with metastatic non-squamous NSCLC with no EGFR or ALK genomic tumor aberrations

• for the treatment of adult patients with metastatic NSCLC who have disease progression during or following platinum-containing chemotherapy. Patients with EGFR or ALK genomic tumor aberrations should have disease progression on FDA-approved therapy for NSCLC harboring these aberrations prior to receiving TECENTRIQ.

Small Cell Lung Cancer (SCLC)

• in combination with carboplatin and etoposide, for the first-line treatment of adult patients with extensive-stage small cell lung cancer (ES-SCLC).

Hepatocellular Carcinoma (HCC)

• in combination with bevacizumab for the treatment of patients with unresectable or metastatic HCC who have not received prior systemic therapy.

Melanoma

• in combination with cobimetinib and vemurafenib for the treatment of patients with BRAF V600 mutation-positive unresectable or metastatic melanoma.

12.1. MECHANISM OF ACTION

PD-L1 may be expressed on tumor cells and/or tumor infiltrating immune cells and can contribute to the inhibition of the anti-tumor immune response in the tumor microenvironment. Binding of PD-L1 to the PD-1 and B7.1 receptors found on T cells and antigen presenting cells suppresses cytotoxic T-cell activity, T-cell proliferation and cytokine production. Atezolizumab is a monoclonal antibody that binds to PD-L1 and blocks its interactions with both PD-1 and B7.1 receptors. This releases the PD-L1/PD-1 mediated inhibition of the immune response, including activation of the anti-tumor immune response without inducing antibodydependent cellular cytotoxicity. In syngeneic mouse tumor models, blocking PD-L1 activity resulted in decreased tumor growth. In mouse models of cancer, dual inhibition of the PD-1/PD-L1 and MAPK pathways suppresses tumor growth and improves tumor immunogenicity through increased antigen presentation and T cell infiltration and activation compared to targeted therapy alone.

DOSAGE AND ADMINISTRATION

Administer TECENTRIQ intravenously over 60 minutes. If the first infusion is tolerated, all subsequent infusions may be delivered over 30 minutes.

Urothelial Carcinoma

• Administer TECENTRIQ as a single agent as 840 mg every 2 weeks, 1200 mg every 3 weeks, or 1680 mg every 4 weeks.

NSCLC

• In the adjuvant setting, administer TECENTRIQ following resection and up to 4 cycles of platinum-based chemotherapy as 840 mg every 2 weeks, 1200 mg every 3 weeks or 1680 mg every 4 weeks for up to 1 year.

• In the metastatic setting, administer TECENTRIQ as 840 mg every 2 weeks, 1200 mg every 3 weeks, or 1680 mg every 4 weeks.

• When administering with chemotherapy with or without bevacizumab, administer TECENTRIQ prior to chemotherapy and bevacizumab when given on the same day.

Small Cell Lung Cancer

• Administer TECENTRIQ as 840 mg every 2 weeks, 1200 mg every 3 weeks, or 1680 mg every 4 weeks. When administering with carboplatin and etoposide, administer TECENTRIQ prior to chemotherapy when given on the same day.

Hepatocellular Carcinoma

• Administer TECENTRIQ as 840 mg every 2 weeks, 1200 mg every 3 weeks, or 1680 mg every 4 weeks. Administer TECENTRIQ prior to bevacizumab when given on the same day. Bevacizumab is administered at 15 mg/kg every 3 weeks.

Melanoma

• Following completion of a 28 day cycle of cobimetinib and vemurafenib, administer TECENTRIQ 840 mg every 2 weeks, 1200 mg every 3 weeks, or 1680 mg every 4 weeks with cobimetinib 60 mg orally once daily (21 days on /7 days off) and vemurafenib 720 mg orally twice daily.

DOSAGE FORMS AND STRENGTHS

Injection: 840 mg/14 mL (60 mg/mL) and 1200 mg/20 mL (60 mg/mL) solution in a single-dose vial.

CONTRAINDICATIONS

None

WARNINGS AND PRECAUTIONS

• Immune-Mediated Adverse Reactions

o Immune-mediated adverse reactions, which may be severe or fatal, can occur in any organ system or tissue, including the following: immune-mediated pneumonitis, immune-mediated colitis, immune-mediated hepatitis, immune-mediated endocrinopathies, immune-mediated dermatologic adverse reactions, immune-mediated nephritis and renal dysfunction, and solid organ transplant rejection.

o Monitor for early identification and management. Evaluate liver enzymes, creatinine, and thyroid function at baseline and periodically during treatment.

o Withhold or permanently discontinue based on severity and type of reaction.

(Further clinical information on these immune-mediated diseases are given in the section on nivolumab)

• Infusion-Related Reactions: Interrupt, slow the rate of infusion, or permanently discontinue based on severity of infusion reactions.

• Complications of Allogeneic HSCT

Fatal and other serious complications can occur in patients who receive allogeneic HSCT before or after being treated with a PD-1/PD-L1 blocking antibody.

• Embryo-Fetal Toxicity

Can cause fetal harm. Advise females of reproductive potential of the potential risk to a fetus and use of effective contraception.

ADVERSE REACTIONS

• Most common adverse reactions (≥ 20%) with TECENTRIQ as a single agent were fatigue/asthenia, decreased appetite, nausea, cough, and dyspnea.

• Most common adverse reactions (≥ 20%) with TECENTRIQ in combination with other antineoplastic drugs in patients with NSCLC and SCLC were fatigue/asthenia, nausea, alopecia, constipation, diarrhea, and decreased appetite.

The most common adverse reactions (≥ 20%) with TECENTRIQ in combination with bevacizumab in patients with HCC were hypertension, fatigue and proteinuria.

• The most common adverse reactions (≥ 20%) with TECENTRIQ in combination with cobimetinib and vemurafenib in patients with melanoma were rash, musculoskeletal pain, fatigue, hepatotoxicity, pyrexia, nausea, pruritus, edema, stomatitis, hypothyroidism, and photosensitivity reaction.

o report SUSPECTED ADVERSE REACTIONS, contact Genentech at 1-888-835-2555 or FDA at 1-800-FDA-1088 or www.fda.gov/medwatch.

USE IN SPECIFIC POPULATIONS

Lactation: advise not to breastfeed.

CLINICAL TRIAL EXPERIENCE

Small Cell Lung Cancer

The efficacy of TECENTRIQ with carboplatin and etoposide was investigated in IMpower133 (NCT02763579), a randomized (1:1), multicenter, double-blind, placebo-controlled trial in 403 patients with extensive stage (ES) SCLC. IMpower133 enrolled patients with ES-SCLC who had received no prior chemotherapy for extensive stage disease and ECOG performance status 0 or 1. The trial excluded patients with active or untreated CNS metastases, history of autoimmune disease, administration of a live, attenuated vaccine within 4 weeks prior to randomization, or administration of systemic immunosuppressive medications within 1 week prior to randomization. Randomization was stratified by sex, ECOG performance status, and presence of brain metastases.

(Figure 53. Histopathology of anaplastic (aka small cell carcinioma, microcellular carcinoma and oat cell carcinoma) carcinoma from the lung)

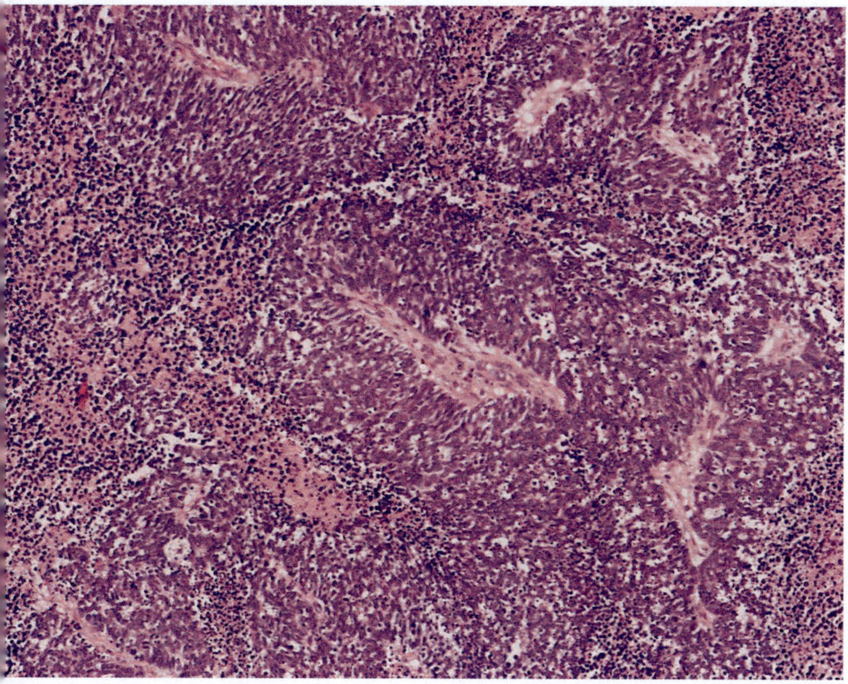

(This image is by Public Domain, https://commons.wikimedia.org/w/index.php?curid=182918; en.wikipedia.org/wiki/Small-cell_carcinoma#/media/File:Carcinoma_microcellulare_oatcell_carcinoma_or_anaplastic_carcinoma_(lung)H&E_magn_200x.jpg. The copyright holder of this work, release this work into the public domain. No changes were made to this image).

Patients were randomized to receive one of the following two treatment arms:

- TECENTRIQ 1200 mg and carboplatin AUC 5 mg/mL/min on Day 1 and etoposide 100 mg/m^2 intravenously on Days 1, 2 and 3 of each 21-day cycle for a maximum of 4 cycles followed by TECENTRIQ 1200 mg once every 3 weeks until disease progression or unacceptable toxicity, or

- placebo and carboplatin AUC 5 mg/mL/min on Day 1 and etoposide 100 mg/m^2 intravenously on Days 1, 2, and 3 of each 21-day cycle for a maximum of 4 cycles followed by placebo once every 3 weeks until disease progression or unacceptable toxicity. Administration of TECENTRIQ was permitted beyond RECIST-defined disease progression. Tumor assessments were conducted every 6 weeks for the first 48 weeks following Cycle 1, Day 1 and then every 9 weeks thereafter. Patients treated beyond disease progression had tumor assessment conducted every 6 weeks until treatment discontinuation.

Major efficacy outcome measures were OS and PFS as assessed by investigator per RECIST v1.1 in the intent-to-treat population. Additional efficacy outcome measures included ORR and DoR as assessed by investigator per RECIST v1.1. A total of 403 patients were randomized, including 201 to the TECENTRIQ arm and 202 to the chemotherapy alone arm. The median age was 64 years (range 26 to 90) and 65% were male. The majority of patients were White (80%); 17% were Asian, 4% were Hispanic and 1% were Black. Baseline ECOG performance status was 0 (35%) or 1 (65%); 9% of patients had a history of brain metastases, and 97% were current or previous smokers.

In the TECENTRIQ with Carboplatin and Etoposide group and the Placebo with Carboplatin and Etoposide group, overall survival was 52% and 66% respectively. The median number of months of progression-free survival was 5.2 and 4.3 months respectively. The objective response rate was 60% and 64% respectively. The median duration of response in months was 4.2 and 3.9 respectively.

6.2. DURVALUMAB (IMFINZI)

INDICATIONS AND USAGE

IMFINZI is a programmed death-ligand 1 (PD-L1) blocking antibody indicated:

- for the treatment of adult patients with unresectable, Stage III **non-small cell lung cancer (NSCLC)** whose disease has not progressed following concurrent platinum-based chemotherapy and radiation therapy.

- in combination with tremelimumab-actl and platinum-based chemotherapy, for the treatment of adult patients with **metastatic non-small cell lung cancer (NSCLC)** with no sensitizing epidermal growth factor receptor (EGFR) mutations or anaplastic lymphoma kinase (ALK) genomic tumor aberrations.

- in combination with etoposide and either carboplatin or cisplatin, as first-line treatment of adult patients with *extensive-stage* ***small cell lung cancer (ES-SCLC)***.

- in combination with gemcitabine and cisplatin, as treatment of adult patients with locally advanced or metastatic **biliary tract cancer (BTC).**

- in combination with tremelimumab-actl, for the treatment of adult patients with unresectable **hepatocellular carcinoma (uHCC).**

12.1. MECHANISM OF ACTION

Expression of programmed cell death ligand-1 (PD-L1) can be induced by inflammatory signals (e.g., IFN-gamma) and can be expressed on both tumor cells and tumor-associated immune cells in the tumor microenvironment. PD-L1 blocks T-cell function and activation through interaction with PD-1 and CD80 (B7.1). By binding to its receptors, PD-L1 reduces cytotoxic T-cell activity, proliferation, and cytokine production. Durvalumab is a human immunoglobulin G1 kappa (IgG1κ) monoclonal antibody that binds to PD-L1 and blocks the interaction of PD-L1 with PD-1 and CD80 (B7.1). Blockade of PD-L1/PD-1 and PD-L1/CD80 interactions releases the inhibition of immune responses, without inducing antibody dependent cell-mediated cytotoxicity (ADCC). PD-L1 blockade with durvalumab led to increased T-cell activation in vitro and decreased tumor size in co-engrafted human tumor and immune cell xenograft mouse models.

DOSAGE AND ADMINISTRATION

- Administer IMFINZI as an intravenous infusion over 60 minutes after dilution.

- Stage III NSCLC:

  o Weight ≥ 30 kg: 10 mg/kg every 2 weeks or 1,500 mg every 4 weeks

  o Weight < 30 kg: 10 mg/kg every 2 weeks

- **Metastatic NSCLC**

  o Weight ≥ 30 kg: 1,500 mg every 3 weeks in combination with tremelimumab-actl 75 mg and platinum-based chemotherapy for 4 cycles, and then administer IMFINZI 1,500 mg every 4 weeks as a single agent with histology-based pemetrexed maintenance therapy every 4 weeks, and a fifth dose of tremelimumab-actl 75 mg in combination with IMFINZI dose 6 at week 16

  o Weight < 30 kg: 20 mg/kg every 3 weeks in combination with tremelimumab-actl 1 mg/kg and platinum-based chemotherapy, and then administer IMFINZI 20 mg/kg every 4 weeks as a single agent with histology-based pemetrexed therapy every 4 weeks, and a fifth dose of tremelimumab-actl 1 mg/kg in combination with IMFINZI dose 6 at week 16 (2.1)

- **ES-SCLC**

  o Weight ≥ 30 kg: with etoposide and either carboplatin or cisplatin, administer IMFINZI 1,500 mg every 3 weeks in combination with chemotherapy, and then 1,500 mg every 4 weeks as a single agent

  o Weight < 30 kg: With etoposide and either carboplatin or cisplatin, administer IMFINZI 20 mg/kg every 3 weeks in combination with chemotherapy, and then 10 mg/kg every 2 weeks as a single agent

- **Biliary tract cancer (BTC)**

  o Weight ≥ 30 kg: administer IMFINZI 1,500 mg every 3 weeks in combination with chemotherapy, and then 1,500 mg every 4 weeks as a single agent

  o Weight < 30 kg: administer IMFINZI 20 mg/kg every 3 weeks in combination with chemotherapy, and then 20 mg/kg every 4 weeks as a single agent

• **Unresectable hepatocellular carcinoma (uHCC)**

o Weight ≥ 30 kg: IMFINZI 1,500 mg in combination with tremelimumab-actl 300 mg as a single dose at Cycle 1/Day 1, followed by IMFINZI as a single agent every 4 weeks

o Weight < 30 kg: IMFINZI 20 mg/kg in combination with tremelimumab-actl 4 mg/kg as a single dose at Cycle 1/Day 1, followed by IMFINZI as a single agent every 4 weeks

DOSAGE FORMS AND STRENGTHS

• Injection: 500 mg/10 mL (50 mg/mL) solution in a single-dose vial.

• Injection: 120 mg/2.4 mL (50 mg/mL) solution in a single-dose vial.

CONTRAINDICATIONS

None

WARNINGS AND PRECAUTIONS

• Immune-Mediated Adverse Reactions

o Immune-mediated adverse reactions, which may be severe or fatal, can occur in any organ system or tissue, including the following: immune-mediated pneumonitis, immune-mediated colitis, immune-mediated hepatitis, immune-mediated endocrinopathies, immune-mediated dermatologic adverse reactions, immunemediated nephritis and renal dysfunction, solid organ transplant rejection, and immune-mediated pancreatitis.

(Further clinical information on the above immune-mediated adverse reactions is given in the section on nivulomab, with the exception of immune-mediated pancreatitis which follows here)

(Immune-mediated pancreatitis is an increasingly recognized type of chronic pancreatitis that can be difficult to distinguish from pancreatic carcinoma but which responds to treatment with corticosteroids, particularly prednisone. Although immune-mediated pancreatitis is quite rare, it constitutes an important clinical problem for both patients and their clinicians: the disease commonly presents itself as a tumorous mass which is diagnostically indistinguishable from pancreatic cancer,

a disease that is much more common in addition to being much more dangerous. Hence, some patients undergo pancreatic surgery, which is associated to substantial mortality and morbidity, out of the fear by patients and clinicians to undertreat a malignancy. However, surgery is not a good treatment for this condition as immune-mediated pancreatitis responds well to immunosuppressive treatment. There are two categories of immune-mediated pancreatitis: Type 1 and Type 2, each with distinct clinical profiles. Type 1 AIP is now regarded as a manifestation of IgG4-related disease, and those affected have tended to be older and to have a high relapse rate.Type 1 pancreatitis, is as such as manifestation of IgG4 disease, which may also affect bile ducts in the liver, salivary glands, kidneys and lymph nodes. Type 2 AIP seems to affect only the pancreas, although about one-third of people with type 2 AIP have associated inflammatory bowel disease. AIP does not affect long-term survival. It is characterized by the following features:

Icterus

Relatively mild symptoms, such as minimal weight loss or nausea.

Increased serum levels of gamma globulins, immunoglobulin G (IgG) or IgG4.

The presence of serum autoantibodies such as anti-nuclear antibody (ANA), anti-lactoferrin antibody, anti-carbonic anhydrase II antibody, and rheumatoid factor (RF).

Contrast-enhanced CT demonstrates a diffusely enlarged (sausage-shaped) pancreas.

Diffuse irregular narrowing of the main pancreatic duct, and stenosis of the intrapancreatic bile duct on endoscopic retrograde cholangiopancreatography (ERCP).

Rare pancreatic calcification or cyst formation.

Marked responsiveness to treatment with corticosteroids).

o Monitor for early identification and management. Evaluate liver enzymes, creatinine, and thyroid function at baseline and periodically during treatment.

o Withhold or permanently discontinue based on severity and type of reaction.

• Infusion-Related Reactions

Interrupt, slow the rate of infusion, or permanently discontinue IMFINZI based on the severity of the reactiion.

• Complications of Allogeneic HSCT: Fatal and other serious complications can occur in patients who receive allogeneic HSCT before or after being treated with a PD-1/PD-L1 blocking antibody.

• Embryo-fetal toxicity: can cause fetal harm. Advise females of reproductive potential of the potential risk to a fetus and use of effective contraception.

ADVERSE REACTIONS

IMFINZI as a Single Agent

• Most common adverse reactions (≥ 20% of patients with unresectable, Stage III NSCLC) are cough, fatigue, pneumonitis/radiation pneumonitis, upper respiratory tract infections, dyspnea, and rash.

IMFINZI in Combination with Platinum-Based Chemotherapy

• Most common adverse reactions (≥ 20% of patients with extensive-stage SCLC) are nausea, fatigue/asthenia, alopecia.

IMFINZI in Combination with gemcitabine and cisplatin

• Most common adverse reactions (≥ 20% of patients with BTC) are fatigue, nausea, constipation, decreased appetite, abdominal pain, rash, and pyrexia.

IMFINZI in Combination with Tremelimumab-actl

• Most common adverse reactions (≥ 20%) of patients with uHCC are rash, diarrhea, fatigue, pruritis, musculoskeletal pain, and abdominal pain.

IMFINZI in Combination with Tremelimumab-actl and Platinum-Based Chemotherapy

• Most common adverse reactions (≥ 20% of patients with metastatic NSCLC) were nausea, fatigue, musculoskeletal pain, decreased appetite, rash, and diarrhea.

To report SUSPECTED ADVERSE REACTIONS, contact AstraZeneca at 1-800-236-9933 or FDA at 1-800-FDA-1088 or www.fda.gov/medwatch.

CLINICAL STUDIES

The experience with IMFENZI's in clinical trials of small cell lung cancer and of biliary tract cancer will be the focus of this section, since the role of other check point inhibitors in other diseases, for which IMFENZI has received FDA approval, has been described earlier in this book.

Small Cell Lung Cancer (SCLC)

The efficacy of IMFINZI in combination with etoposide and either carboplatin or cisplatin in previously untreated ES-SCLC was investigated in CASPIAN, a randomized, multicenter, active-controlled, openlabel trial (NCT03043872). Eligible patients had WHO Performance Status of 0 or 1 and were suitable to receive a platinum-based chemotherapy regimen as first-line treatment for SCLC. Patients with asymptomatic or treated brain metastases were eligible. Choice of platinum agent was at the investigator's discretion, taking into consideration the calculated creatinine clearance. Patients with history of chest radiation therapy; a history of active primary immunodeficiency; autoimmune disorders including paraneoplastic syndrome; active or prior documented autoimmune or inflammatory disorders; use of systemic immunosuppressants within 14 days before the first dose of the treatment except physiological dose of systemic corticosteroids were ineligible.

Randomization was stratified by the planned platinum-based therapy in cycle 1 (carboplatin or cisplatin).

The evaluation of efficacy for ES-SCLC relied on comparison between: IMFINZI 1,500 mg, and investigator's choice of carboplatin (AUC 5 or 6 mg/mL/min) or cisplatin (75-80 mg/m^2) on Day 1 and etoposide (80-100 mg/m^2) intravenously on Days 1, 2, and 3 of each 21-day cycle for 4 cycles, followed by IMFINZI 1,500 mg every 4 weeks until disease progression or unacceptable toxicity, or Investigator's choice of carboplatin (AUC 5 or 6 mg/mL/min) or cisplatin (75-80 mg/m^2) on Day 1 and etoposide (80-100 mg/m^2) intravenously on Days 1, 2, and 3 of each 21-day cycle, up to 6 cycles. After completion of chemotherapy, prophylactic cranial irradiation (PCI) was administered per investigator discretion. Administration of IMFINZI as a single agent was permitted beyond disease progression if the patient was clinically stable and deriving clinical benefit as determined by the investigator. The major efficacy outcome measure was overall survival (OS) of IMFINZI plus chemotherapy vs. chemotherapy alone. Additional efficacy outcome measures were investigator-assessed progression-free survival (PFS) and objective response rate (ORR), per RECIST v1.1.

The study population characteristics were: median age of 63 years (range: 28 to 82); 40% age 65 or older; 70% male; 84% White, 15% Asian, and 0.9% Black; 65% WHO/ECOG PS of 1; and 93% were former/current smokers. Ninety percent of patients had Stage IV disease and 10% had brain metastasis at baseline. A total of 25% of the patients received cisplatin and 74% of the patients received carboplatin. In the chemotherapy alone arm, 57% of the patients received 6 cycles of chemotherapy, and 8% of the patients received PCI.

The median overall survival in months of patients who received IMFINZI with Etoposide and either Carboplatin or Cisplatin (n=268) versus those who received Etoposide and either Carboplatin or Cisplatin (n=269) was 13.0 and 10.3 respectively. The Hazard ratio was 0.73 and the p-value was 0.0047.

Biliary Tract Cancer (BTC)

The efficacy of IMFINZI in combination with gemcitabine and cisplatin in patients with locally advanced or metastatic BTC was investigated in TOPAZ-1 (NCT03875235), a randomized, double-blind, placebo-controlled, multicenter trial that enrolled 685 patients with histologically confirmed locally advanced unresectable or metastatic BTC who have not previously received systemic therapy. Patients with recurrent disease > 6 months after surgery and/or completion of adjuvant therapy were eligible. Patients had an ECOG Performance status of 0 and 1 and at least one target lesion by RECIST 1.1. Patients with ampullary carcinoma; active or prior documented autoimmune or inflammatory disorders; HIV infection or active infections, including tuberculosis or hepatitis C; current or prior use of immunosuppressive medication within 14 days before the first dose of IMFINZI were ineligible.

Randomization was stratified by disease status (recurrent vs. initially unresectable) and primary tumor location (intrahepatic cholangiocarcinoma [ICCA] vs. extrahepatic cholangiocarcinoma [ECCA] vs. gallbladder cancer [GBC]).

Patients were randomized 1:1 to receive

- IMFINZI 1,500 mg on Day 1+ gemcitabine 1,000 mg/m^2 and cisplatin 25 mg/m^2 on Days 1 and 8 of each 21-day cycle up to 8 cycles, followed by IMFINZI 1,500 mg every 4 weeks, or

- Placebo on Day 1+ gemcitabine 1,000 mg/m^2 and cisplatin 25 mg/m^2 on Days 1 and 8 of each 21-day cycle up to 8 cycles, followed by placebo every 4 weeks.

Treatment with IMFINZI or placebo continued until disease progression, or unacceptable toxicity. Treatment beyond disease progression was permitted if the patient was clinically stable and deriving clinical benefit as determined by the investigator.

The major efficacy outcome measure was overall survival (OS). Additional efficacy outcome measures were investigator-assessed progression-free survival (PFS), objective response rate (ORR) and duration of response (DoR). Tumor assessments were conducted every 6 weeks for the first 24 weeks after the date of randomization, and then every 8 weeks until confirmed objective disease progression.

The study population characteristics were: 50% male, median age of 64 years (range 20-85), 47% age 65 or older; 56% Asian, 37% White, 2% Black or African American, 0.1% American Indian or Alaskan Native, and 4% other; 51% had an ECOG PS of 1; primary tumor location was ICCA 56%, ECCA 18% and GBC 25%; 20% of patients had recurrent disease; 86% of patients had metastatic and 14% had locally advanced disease.

At a pre-specified interim analysis, the trial demonstrated a statistically significant improvement in OS and PFS in patients randomized to IMFINZI in combination with chemotherapy compared to placebo in combination with chemotherapy.

6.3. AVELUMAB (BAVENCIO®)

Initial U.S. Approval: 2017

RECENT MAJOR CHANGES

INDICATIONS AND USAGE

BAVENCIO is a programmed death ligand-1 (PD-L1) blocking antibody indicated for:

Merkel Cell Carcinoma (MCC) *(MCC is also known as primary neuroendocrine carcinoma of the skin, primary small cell carcinoma of the skin, and trabecular carcinoma of the skin).*

(Figure 54. Mitosis in a neuroendocrine tumor)

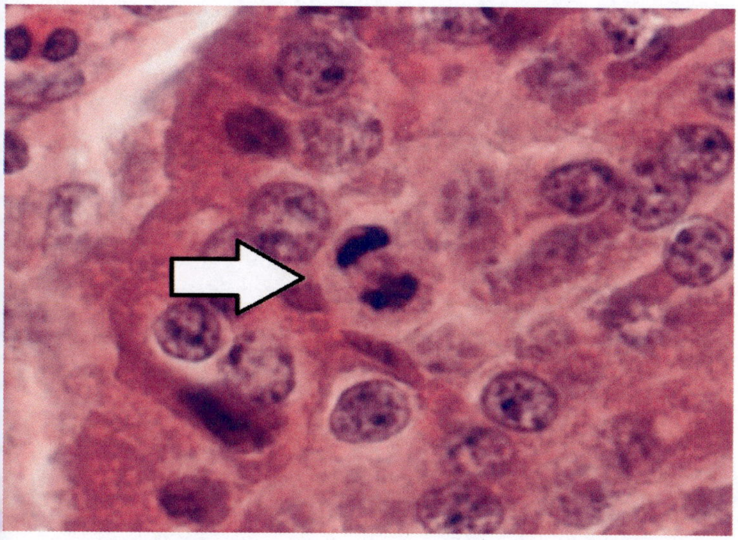

(This image is by Mikael Häggström, M.D. - Own work, CC0, https://commons.wikimedia.org/w/index.php?curid=86416413; https://en.wikipedia.org/wiki/Neuroendocrine_tumor#/media/File:Mitosis_in_a_neuroendocrine_tumor.jpg. This file is made available under the Creative Commons CC0 1.0 Universal Public Domain Dedication. No changes were made to this image).

(Factors involved in the development of MCC include the Merkel cell polyomavirus [MCV]).

• Adults and pediatric patients 12 years and older with **metastatic MCC**. This indication is approved under accelerated approval based on tumor response rate and duration of response. Continued approval for this indication may be contingent upon verification and description of clinical benefit in confirmatory trials.

Urothelial Carcinoma (UC)

• Maintenance treatment of patients with locally advanced or metastatic UC that has not progressed with first-line platinum-containing chemotherapy.

• Patients with locally advanced or metastatic UC who

• Have disease progression during or following platinum-containing chemotherapy.

Have disease progression within 12 months of neoadjuvant or adjuvant treatment with platinum-containing chemotherapy

Renal Cell Carcinoma (RCC)

• First-line treatment, in combination with axitinib, of patients with advanced RCC.

12.1. MECHANISM OF ACTION

PD-L1 may be expressed on tumor cells and tumor-infiltrating immune cells and can contribute to the inhibition of the anti-tumor immune response in the tumor microenvironment. Binding of PD-L1 to the PD-1 and B7.1 receptors found on T cells and antigen presenting cells suppresses cytotoxic T-cell activity, T-cell proliferation, and cytokine production. Avelumab binds PD-L1 and blocks the interaction between PD-L1 and its receptors PD-1 and B7.1. This interaction releases the inhibitory effects of PD-L1 on the immune response resulting in the restoration of immune responses, including anti-tumor immune responses. Avelumab has also been shown to induce antibody-dependent cell-mediated cytotoxicity (ADCC) in vitro. In syngeneic mouse tumor models, blocking PD-L1 activity resulted in decreased tumor growth.

DOSAGE AND ADMINISTRATION

• Premedicate for the first 4 infusions and subsequently as needed

• Merkel Cell Carcinoma: 800 mg every 2 weeks

• Urothelial Carcinoma; 800 mg every 2 weeks

Renal Cell Carcinoma: 800 mg every 2 weeks in combination with axitinib 5 mg orally twice daily.

Administer BAVENCIO as an intravenous infusion over 60 minutes

DOSAGE FORMS AND STRENGTHS

Injection: 200 mg/10 mL (20 mg/mL) solution in single-dose vial
(CONTRAINDICATIONS

None

WARNINGS AND PRECAUTIONS

• Immune-mediated pneumonitis

Withhold for moderate pneumonitis; permanently discontinue for severe, life-threatening, or recurrent moderate pneumonitis

• Hepatotoxicity and immune-mediated hepatitis

Monitor for changes in liver function. Withhold for moderate hepatitis; permanently discontinue for severe or life-threatening hepatitis

• Immune-mediated colitis

Withhold for moderate or severe colitis; permanently discontinue for life-threatening or recurrent severe colitis.

Immune-mediated endocrinopathies

Withhold for severe or life-threatening endocrinopathies

• Immune-mediated nephritis and renal dysfunction

Withhold for moderate or severe nephritis and renal dysfunction; permanently discontinue for life threatening nephritis or renal dysfunction

(Further clinical information on these immune-mediated disorders is given in the section on nivolumab).

• Infusion-related reactions

Interrupt or slow the rate of infusion for mild or moderate infusion-related reactions. Stop the infusion and permanently discontinue BAVENCIO for severe or life-threatening infusion-related reactions.

• Major adverse cardiovascular events

Optimize management of cardiovascular risk factors. Discontinue BAVENCIO in combination with axitinib for Grade 3-4 events.

• Embryo-fetal toxicity

BAVENCIO can cause fetal harm. Advise of potential risk to a fetus and use of effective contraception.

ADVERSE REACTIONS

Most common adverse reactions (> 20%) in patients were:

• MCC: fatigue, musculoskeletal pain, diarrhea, nausea, infusion-related reaction, rash, decreased appetite, and peripheral edema.

• UC: • Maintenance treatment: fatigue, musculoskeletal pain, urinary tract infection, and rash.

• Previously-treated: fatigue, infusion-related reaction, musculoskeletal pain, nausea, decreased appetite, and urinary tract infection.

• RCC (with axitinib): diarrhea, fatigue, hypertension, musculoskeletal pain, nausea, mucositis, palmar-plantar erythrodysesthesia, dysphonia, decreased appetite, hypothyroidism, rash, hepatotoxicity, cough, dyspnea, abdominal pain, and headache.

To report SUSPECTED ADVERSE REACTIONS, contact EMD Serono at 1-800-283-8088 ext. 5563 or FDA at 1-800-FDA-1088 or www.fda.gov/medwatch.

USE IN SPECIFIC POPULATIONS

Lactation: advise not to breastfeed

CLINICAL TRIAL EXPERIENCE

Since Bavencio is only one of two check point inhibitors active in Merkel's carcinoma, only clinical trial information for this disease will be presented here.

Metastatic Merkel Cell Carcinoma

The efficacy and safety of BAVENCIO was demonstrated in the JAVELIN Merkel 200 trial (NCT02155647), an open-label, single-arm, multi-center study conducted in patients with histologically confirmed metastatic MCC whose disease had progressed on or after chemotherapy administered for distant metastatic disease. The trial excluded patients with autoimmune disease; medical conditions requiring systemic immunosuppression; prior organ or allogeneic stem cell transplantation; prior treatment with anti-PD-1, anti-PD-L1, or anti-CTLA-4 antibodies; CNS metastases; infection with HIV, hepatitis B, or hepatitis C; or ECOG performance score ≥ 2.

Patients received BAVENCIO 10 mg/kg as an intravenous infusion over 60 minutes every 2 weeks until disease progression or unacceptable toxicity. Patients with radiological disease progression not associated with significant clinical deterioration, defined as no new or worsening symptoms, no change in performance status for greater than 2 weeks, and no need for salvage therapy, could continue treatment. Tumor response assessments were performed every 6 weeks.

The major efficacy outcome measures were confirmed overall response rate (ORR) according to Response Evaluation Criteria in Solid Tumors (RECIST) v1.1 as assessed by a blinded independent central review committee (IRC) and IRC-assessed duration of response. The efficacy analysis was conducted when the last patient enrolled had completed 12 months of follow-up. A total of 88 patients were enrolled. Baseline patient characteristics were a median age of 73 years (range: 33 to 88), 74% of patients were male, 92% were White, and the ECOG performance score was 0 (56%) or 1 (44%). Seventy-five percent of patients were 65 years or older, 35% were 75 or older, and 3% were 85 or older. Sixty-five percent of patients were reported to have had one prior anti-cancer therapy for metastatic MCC and 35% had two or more prior therapies. Fifty-three percent of patients had visceral metastases.

All patients had tumor samples evaluated for PD-L1 expression; of these, 66% were PD-L1-positive (≥ 1% of tumor cells), 18% were PD-L1 negative, and 16% had non-evaluable results by an investigational immunohistochemistry assay. Archival tumor samples were evaluated for Merkel cell polyomavirus (MCV) using an investigational assay; of the 77 patients with evaluable results, 52% had evidence of MCV. Responses were observed in patients regardless of tumor PD-L1 expression or presence of MCV.

The overall response rate was 33% with a complete response in 11.4% and a partial response in 21.6%. The duration of response was 2.8 to 23.3+ months.

7. CTLA-4 inhibitors

7.1. Ipilumumab (YERVOY)

YERVOY® (ipilimumab) injection, for intravenous use.

Initial U.S. Approval: 2011

BOXED WARNING: IMMUNE-MEDIATED ADVERSE REACTIONS See full prescribing information for complete boxed warning. YERVOY can result in severe and fatal immune-mediated adverse reactions. These immune-mediated reactions may involve any organ system; however, the most common severe immune-mediated adverse reactions are enterocolitis, hepatitis, dermatitis (including toxic epidermal necrolysis), neuropathy, and endocrinopathy. The majority of these immune-mediated reactions initially manifested during treatment; however, a minority occurred weeks to months after discontinuation of YERVOY. Permanently discontinue YERVOY and initiate systemic high-dose corticosteroid therapy for severe immune-mediated reactions. Assess patients for signs and symptoms of enterocolitis, dermatitis, neuropathy, and endocrinopathy and evaluate clinical chemistries including liver function tests, adrenocorticotropic hormone (ACTH) level, and thyroid function tests at baseline and before each dose.

YERVOY is a human cytotoxic T-lymphocyte antigen 4 (CTLA-4)-blocking antibody indicated for:

- Treatment of unresectable or metastatic **melanoma** in adults and pediatric patients (12 years and older).

- Adjuvant treatment of patients with cutaneous **melanoma** with pathologic involvement of regional lymph nodes of more than 1 mm who have undergone complete resection, including total lymphadenectomy.

- Treatment of patients with intermediate or poor risk, previously untreated advanced **renal cell carcinoma**, in combination with nivolumab.

- Treatment of adult and pediatric patients 12 years of age and older with **microsatellite instability-high (MSI-H) or mismatch repair deficient (dMMR) metastatic colorectal cancer** that has progressed following treatment with a fluoropyrimidine, oxaliplatin, and irinotecan, in combination with nivolumab. This indication is approved under accelerated approval based on overall response rate and duration of response. Continued approval for this indication may be contingent upon verification and description of clinical benefit in confirmatory trials.

12.1 MECHANISM OF ACTION

CTLA-4 is a negative regulator of T-cell activation. Ipilimumab binds to CTLA-4 and blocks the interaction of CTLA-4 with its ligands, CD80/CD86. Blockade of CTLA-4 has been shown to augment T-cell activation and proliferation. The mechanism of action of ipilimumab's effect in patients with melanoma is indirect, possibly through T-cell mediated anti-tumor immune responses.

(Figure 55. Space-filling model of the Fab fragment of the monoclonal antibody ipilimumab (blue) bound to its target, CTLA-4 (pale green). Style made to resemble the Protein Data Bank's "Molecule of the Month" series, illustrated by Dr. David S. Goodsell of the Scripps Research Institute).

(This image is by Fvasconcellos - Public Domain, https://commons.wikimedia.org/w/index.php?curid=61347389; https://en.wikipedia.org/wiki/Ipilimumab#/media/File:Ipilimumab_5TRU.png. The copyright holder of this work, release this work into the public domain. No changes were made to this image).

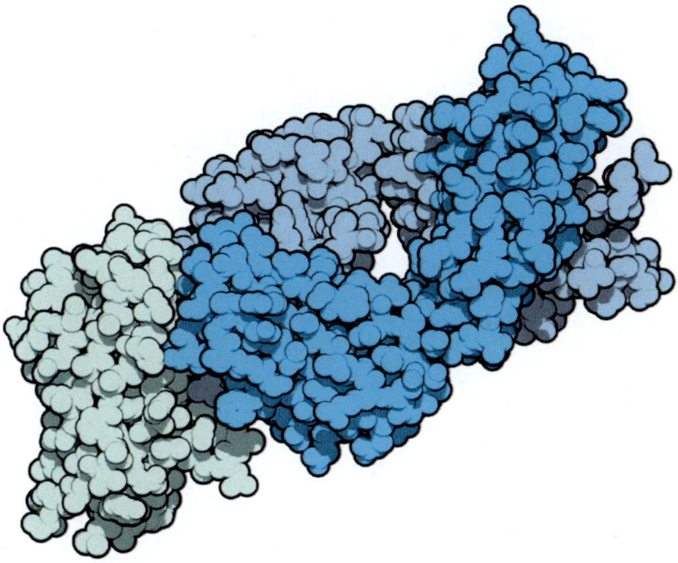

DOSAGE AND ADMINISTRATION

- Unresectable or metastatic melanoma

o YERVOY 3 mg/kg administered intravenously over 90 minutes every 3 weeks for a total of 4 doses.

- Adjuvant melanoma

o YERVOY 10 mg/kg administered intravenously over 90 minutes every 3 weeks for 4 doses, followed by 10 mg/kg every 12 weeks for up to 3 years or until documented disease recurrence or unacceptable toxicity

- Advanced renal cell carcinoma

o Nivolumab 3 mg/kg administered intravenously over 30 minutes followed by YERVOY 1 mg/kg administered intravenously over 30 minutes on the same day, every 3 weeks for 4 doses, then nivolumab 240 mg every 2 weeks or 480 mg every 4 weeks, administered intravenously over 30 minutes.

Microsatellite instability-high (MSI-H) or mismatch repair deficient (dMMR) metastatic colorectal cancer

o Nivolumab 3 mg/kg followed by YERVOY 1 mg/kg on the same day every 3 weeks for 4 doses, then nivolumab 240 mg every 2 weeks

- Permanently discontinue for severe adverse reactions.

DOSAGE FORMS AND STRENGTHS

Injection: 50 mg/10 mL (5 mg/mL) and 200 mg/40 mL (5 mg/mL) in a single use vial.

CONTRAINDICATIONS

None.

WARNINGS AND PRECAUTIONS

Immune-mediated adverse reactions: Permanently discontinue for severe reactions. Withhold dose for moderate immune-mediated adverse reactions until return to baseline, improvement to mild severity, or complete resolution, and patient is receiving less than 7.5 mg prednisone or equivalent per day. Administer systemic high-dose corticosteroids for severe, persistent, or recurring immune-mediated reactions.

• Immune-mediated hepatitis: Evaluate liver function tests before each dose of YERVOY. Withhold for moderate and permanently discontinue for severe or life-threatening transaminase or total bilirubin elevation.

• Immune-mediated endocrinopathies

Monitor clinical chemistries, ACTH level, and thyroid function tests prior to each dose. Evaluate at each visit for signs and symptoms of endocrinopathy. Institute hormone replacement therapy as needed.

• Immune-mediated pneumonitis

Withhold for moderate and permanently discontinue for severe or life-threatening pneumonitis.

• Immune-mediated nephritis and renal dysfunction

Monitor for changes in renal function. Withhold for moderate or severe and permanently discontinue for life-threatening serum creatinine elevation.

• Immune-mediated encephalitis

Monitor for changes in neurologic function. Withhold for new-onset moderate to severe neurological signs or symptoms and permanently discontinue for immune-mediated encephalitis.

(Further clinical information on immune-mediated complications of check point inhibitors is given in the section on nivolumab)

• Infusion reactions: Discontinue for severe and life-threatening infusion reactions. Interrupt or slow the rate of infusion in patients with mild or moderate infusion reactions.

• Embryo-Fetal toxicity

Can cause fetal harm. Advise of potential risk to a fetus and use of effective contraception.

ADVERSE REACTIONS

Most common adverse reactions (≥5%) with YERVOY as a single agent are fatigue, diarrhea, pruritus, rash, and colitis. Additional common adverse reactions at the 10 mg/kg dose (≥5%) include nausea, vomiting, headache, weight loss, pyrexia, decreased appetite, and insomnia.

Most common adverse reactions (≥20%) with YERVOY in combination with nivolumab are fatigue, rash, diarrhea, nausea, pyrexia, musculoskeletal pain, pruritus, abdominal pain, vomiting, cough, arthralgia, decreased appetite, dyspnea.

To report SUSPECTED ADVERSE REACTIONS, contact Bristol-Myers Squibb at 1-800-721-5072 or FDA at 1-800-FDA-1088 or www.fda.gov/medwatch.

USE IN SPECIFIC POPULATIONS

- Lactation: Discontinue breastfeeding during treatment with YERVOY.

14. CLINICAL STUDIES

14.3 Overall Survival Previously Untreated Advanced Renal Cell Carcinoma

Yervoy is FDA-approved for use in renal cell carcinoma, unlike most other check point inhibitors, so this book will focus on the clinical trial experience in this indication

CHECKMATE-214 (NCT02231749) was a randomized (1:1), open-label study in patients with previously untreated advanced RCC. Patients were included regardless of their PD-L1 status. CHECKMATE-214 excluded patients with any history of or concurrent brain metastases, active autoimmune disease, or medical conditions requiring systemic immunosuppression. Patients were stratified by International Metastatic RCC Database Consortium (IMDC) prognostic score and region.

Efficacy was evaluated in intermediate/poor risk patients with at least 1 or more of 6 prognostic risk factors as per the IMDC criteria (less than one year from time of initial renal cell carcinoma diagnosis to randomization, Karnofsky performance status <80%, hemoglobin less than the lower limit of normal, corrected calcium of greater than 10 mg/dL, platelet count greater than the upper limit of normal, and absolute neutrophil count greater than the upper limit of normal.

Patients were randomized to nivolumab 3 mg/kg plus YERVOY 1 mg/kg (n=425) administered intravenously every 3 weeks for 4 doses followed by nivolumab monotherapy 3 mg/kg every two weeks or to sunitinib (n=422) administered orally 50 mg daily for 4 weeks followed by 2 weeks off, every cycle. Treatment continued until disease progression or unacceptable toxicity. The median age was 61 years (range: 21 to 85) with 38% ≥65 years of age and 8% ≥75 years of age. The majority of patients were male (73%) and white (87%) and 26% and 74% of patients had a baseline KPS of 70% to 80% and 90% to 100%, respectively.

The major efficacy outcome measures were OS, PFS (IRRC-assessed), and confirmed ORR (IRRC-assessed) in intermediate/poor risk patients. In this population, the trial demonstrated statistically significant improvement in OS and ORR for patients randomized to nivolumab plus YERVOY as compared with sunitinib. OS benefit was observed regardless of PD-L1 expression level. The trial did not demonstrate a statistically significant improvement in PFS.

Confirmed objective response in nivolumab plus YERVOY versus the sunitinib group was 41.6% versus 26.5% respectively, p-value 0.0001. The complete response rate was 40% versus 5% respectively. The median progression-free survival was 11.6 versus 8.4 months respectively. The hazard ratio 0.82; the p-value was not significant at alpha level of 0.009

7.2. Tremelimumab/IMJUDO

IMJUDO® (tremelimumab-actl) injection, for intravenous use Initial U.S. Approval: 2022

INDICATIONS AND USAGE

IMJUDO is a cytotoxic T-lymphocyte-associated antigen 4 (CTLA-4) blocking antibody indicated in combination with durvalumab, for the treatment of adult patients with **unresectable hepatocellular carcinoma (uHCC).**

12.1 MECHANISM OF ACTION

CTLA-4 is a negative regulator of T-cell activity. Tremelimumab-actl is a monoclonal antibody that binds to CTLA-4 and blocks the interaction with its ligands CD80 and CD86, releasing CTLA-4-mediated inhibition of T-cell activation. In synergistic mouse tumor models, blocking CTLA-4 activity resulted in decreased tumor growth and increased proliferation of T cells in tumors.

DOSAGE AND ADMINISTRATION

• Administer IMJUDO as an intravenous infusion over 60 minutes after dilution.

o Weight 30 kg and more: IMJUDO 300 mg as a single dose in combination with durvalumab 1,500 mg at Cycle 1/Day 1, followed by durvalumab as a single agent every 4 weeks

o Weight less than 30 kg: IMJUDO 4 mg/kg as a single dose in combination with durvalumab 20 mg/kg at Cycle 1/Day 1, followed by durvalumab as a single agent every 4 weeks instructions and dosage modifications for adverse reactions

FORMS AND STRENGTHS

• Injection: 25 mg/1.25 mL (20 mg/mL) solution in a single-dose vial.

Injection: 300 mg/15 mL (20 mg/mL) solution in a single-dose vial.

CONTRAINDICATIONS

None

WARNINGS AND PRECAUTIONS

• Immune-Mediated Adverse Reactions

o Immune-mediated adverse reactions, which may be severe or fatal, can occur in any organ system or tissue, including the following: immune-mediated pneumonitis, immune-mediated colitis, immune-mediated hepatitis, immune-mediated endocrinopathies, immune-mediated dermatologic adverse reactions, immune mediated nephritis with renal dysfunction and immune-mediated pancreatitis.

o Monitor for early identification and management. Evaluate liver enzymes, creatinine, adrenocorticotropic hormone level and thyroid function at baseline and before each dose.

o Withhold or permanently discontinue based on severity and type of reaction.

(Further clinical information on immune-mediated disorders due to check point inhibitor treatment is give in the section on nivolumab).

• Infusion-Related Reactions

Interrupt, slow the rate of infusion, or permanently discontinue treatment based on the severity of the reaction.

Embryo-fetal toxicity

Can cause fetal harm. Advise females of reproductive potential of the potential risk to a fetus and use of effective contraception.

ADVERSE REACTIONS

Most common adverse reactions (≥ 20%) of patients with uHCC are rash, diarrhea, fatigue, pruritus, musculoskeletal pain, and abdominal pain.

Most common laboratory abnormalities (≥ 40%) of patients with uHCC are AST increased, ALT increased, hemoglobin decreased, sodium decreased, bilirubin increased, alkaline phosphatase increased, and lymphocytes decreased.

To report SUSPECTED ADVERSE REACTIONS, contact AstraZeneca at 1-800-236-9933 or FDA at 1-800-FDA-1088 or www.fda.gov/medwatch.

USE IN SPECIFIC POPULATIONS

Lactation: Advise not to breastfeed

14. CLINICAL STUDIES

14.1 Unresectable Hepatocellular Carcinoma (HCC)

The efficacy of IMJUDO in combination with durvalumab was evaluated in the HIMALAYA study (NCT03298451), a randomized (1:1:1), open-label, multicenter study in patients with confirmed uHCC who had not received prior systemic treatment for HCC. Patients were randomized as follows: IMJUDO plus durvalumab or durvalumab, or sorafenib.

Study treatment consisted of

- IMJUDO as a one-time single intravenous infusion of 300 mg in combination with durvalumab 1,500 mg on the same day, followed by durvalumab every 4 weeks
- durvalumab 1,500 mg every 4 weeks (an unapproved regimen for uHCC) or

- sorafenib 400 mg given orally twice daily, until disease progression or unacceptable toxicity.

The efficacy assessment of IMJUDO is based on patients randomized to the IMJUDO plus durvalumab arm versus the sorafenib arm. Randomization was stratified by macrovascular invasion (MVI) (yes or no), etiology of liver disease (hepatitis B virus vs. hepatitis C virus vs. others) and ECOG performance status (0 vs. 1). The study enrolled patients with Barcelona Clinic Liver Cancer (BCLC) Stage C or B (not eligible for locoregional therapy). The study excluded patients with co-infection of viral hepatitis B and hepatitis C; active or prior documented gastrointestinal (GI) bleeding within 12 months; ascites requiring non-pharmacologic intervention within 6 months; hepatic encephalopathy within 12 months before the start of treatment; active or prior documented autoimmune or inflammatory disorders. Esophagogastroduodenoscopy was not mandated prior to enrollment but adequate endoscopic therapy, according to institutional standards, was required for patients with a history of esophageal variceal bleeding or those assessed as high risk for esophageal variceal bleeding by the treating physician. Study treatment was permitted beyond disease progression if the patient was clinically stable and was deriving clinical benefit as determined by the investigator.

The major efficacy outcome measure was overall survival (OS) between the IMJUDO plus durvalumab arm versus the sorafenib arm. Additional efficacy outcomes were investigator-assessed progression-free survival (PFS), objective response rate (ORR) and duration of response (DoR) according to RECIST v1.1. Tumor assessments were conducted every 8 weeks for the first 12 months and then every 12 weeks thereafter. The baseline demographics of the IMJUDO plus durvalumab and sorafenib arms were as follows: male (85%), age < 65 years (50%), median age of 65 years (range: 18 to 88 years), White (46%), Asian (49%), Black or African American (2%), Native Hawaiian or other Pacific Islander (0.1%), race Unknown (2%), Hispanic or Latino (5%), Not Hispanic or Latino (94%), ethnicity Unknown (1%), ECOG PS 0 (62%); Child-Pugh Class score A (99%), macrovascular invasion (26%), extrahepatic spread (53%), viral etiology hepatitis B (31%), hepatitis C (27%), uninfected (42%).

The median overall survival between the IMJUDO and durvalumab group versus the sorafenib group was 16.4 versus 13.8 months respectively. The hazard ratio was 0.78 and the p-value was 0.0035. The median progression-free survival was 3.8 and 4.1 months respectively.

8. CONCLUSIONS

The efficacy of check point inhibitors is astonishing. Major improvements have been made by them: advanced melanoma is probably the best example. Additionally, some advanced solid tumors for which there was little or no effective treatment now have a treatment option: unresectable hepatic cell carcinoma, metastatic pancreatic carcinoma, advanced adrenocortical carcinoma are examples. Some of these results were obtained using a check point inhibitor in combination with cytotoxic chemotherapy appropriate for the disease in question, while other results were obtained using a combination of check point inhibitors. The future is promising. What a great time to be practicing medical oncology with not only check point inhibitor therapies but tyrosine kinase inhibitors and chimeric antigen reactive (CAR) T cells all becoming available.

REFERENCES

1. Shiravand Y, Khodadadi F, Kashani SMA, Hosseini-Fard SR, Hosseini S, Sadeghirad H, Ladwa R, O'Byrne K, Kulasinghe A. Immune Check point inhibitors in Cancer Therapy. Curr Oncol. 2022 Apr 24;29(5):3044-3060. doi: 10.3390/curroncol29050247. PMID: 35621637; PMCID: PMC9139602.

2.Kennedy R, Awada H, Vura N, Ciltea D, Morocco M. Endocrinopathies from check point inhibitors: Incidence, outcomes, and management. Cleveland Clin J Med. 2023 May 1;90(5):307-317. doi: 10.3949/ccjm.90a.22032. PMID: 37127339.

3.Twomey, Julianne D., and Baolin Zhang. Cancer immunotherapy update: FDA-approved check point inhibitors and companion diagnostics. *The AAPS journal* 23 (2021): 1-11.

4.Barroso-Sousa R, Barry WT, Garrido-Castro AC, Hodi FS, Min L, Krop IE, Tolaney SM. Incidence of Endocrine Dysfunction Following the Use of Different Immune

Check point inhibitor Regimens: A Systematic Review and Meta-analysis. JAMA Oncol. 2018 Feb 1;4(2):173-182. doi: 10.1001/jamaoncol.2017.3064. PMID: 28973656; PMCID: PMC5838579.

5.Geisler AN, Phillips GS, Barrios DM, Wu J, Leung DYM, Moy AP, Kern JA, Lacouture ME. Immune check point inhibitor-related dermatologic adverse events. J Am Acad Dermatol. 2020 Nov;83(5):1255-1268. doi: 10.1016/j.jaad.2020.03.132. Epub 2020 May 23. PMID: 32454097; PMCID: PMC7572894.

6.Palaskas N, Lopez-Mattei J, Durand JB, Iliescu C, Deswal A. Immune Check point inhibitor Myocarditis: Pathophysiological Characteristics, Diagnosis, and Treatment. J Am Heart Assoc. 2020 Jan 21;9(2):e013757. doi: 10.1161/JAHA.119.013757. Epub 2020 Jan 21. PMID: 31960755; PMCID: PMC7033840.

ABBREVIATIONS USED

Abbreviations used (other than those explained in the FDA Highlights of Prescribing and the FDA Full Prescribing Information) are listed below. This list includes abbreviations used in other books in the series Medicine 2020 and the series Modern Medicine.

AC, adriamycin and cyclophosphamide (combination chemotherapy)

ACE, angiotensin-converting-enzyme

ADC, antibody-drug conjugate

ADCC, antibody-dependent cellular cytotoxicity

ADCC, antibody directed enzyme prodrug therapy

AGEP, acute generalized exanthematous pustulosis

AI, aromatase inhibitor

ALK, anaplastic lymphoma kinase

ALL, acute lymphoblastic leukemia

ALT, alanine aminotransferase

AML, acute myeloid leukemia

aPTT, activated partial thromboplastin time

ARR, administration-related reaction

AS, adverse reaction

AS, ankylosing spondylitis

ASCT, autologous stem cell transplant

AST, aspartate aminotransferase

ATA, anti-therapeutic antibody

ATM, ataxia telangiectasia mutated (gene)

AUC, Area Under the Concentration – time curve

AUC (0-inf): AUC curve to infinite time. As we cannot get the assays to go to infinity, we have to extrapolate to infinity. This can be calculated from the AUC(0-t) by the addition of a constant (Clast/λz), where Clast is the last observed quantifiable concentration and λz is the terminal phase rate constant.

BCG, Bacille Calmain-Guerin

BCMA, B cell maturation antigen

BCR-ABL, breakpoint cluster region/Abelson

BCRP, breast cancer resistance protein

BIRC, blinded independent review committee

b DMARD, biologic disease-modifying anti-rheumatic drug

BRACA1, breast cancer susceptibility gene 1

BTK, Bruton's tyrosine kinase

CAT, cyclophosphamide, adriamycin and taxane (combination chemotherapy)

CDC, complement-dependent cytotoxicity

CDK, cyclin-dependent kinase

C-G, Cockroft-Gault (formula)

cHL, classical Hodgkin Lymphoma

CINV, chemotherapy-induced nausea and vomiting

CIS, carcinoma in situ

CLL, chronic lymphocytic leukemia

Clcr, creatinine clearance rate

CMF, cyclophosphamide, methotrexate, and fluorouracil (combination chemotherapy

CML, chronic myelogenous leukemia (also known as chronic myeloid leukemia)

CPS, combine positive score

CR, complete remission

CRC, colorectal carcinoma

CRISPR, clustered regulatory interspaced short palindromic repeats

CRS, cytokine release syndrome

CS, cytokine storm

csDMARD, synthetic disease-modifying anti-rheumatic drug

CSF1R, colony-stimulating factor receptor 1

CT, computed tomography

CTCAE, Common Terminology Criteria for Adverse Events

CVVHD, continuous veno-venous hemodialysis

DBCL, diffuse B cell lymphoma

DCIS, ductal carcinoma in situ

DFS, disease-free survival

dMMR, deficient mismatch repair

DLBCL, diffuse large B cell lymphoma

DMSO, dimethyl sulfoxide

DoR, duration of remission

DPP4, dipeptidyl peptidase-4

DRESS, drug reaction with eosinophilia and systemic symptoms. DRESS syndrome is classified as one form of severe cutaneous adverse reactions (SCARs). In addition to DRESS, SCARs includes four other drug-induced skin reactions, the Stevens–Johnson syndrome (SJS); Toxic epidermal necrolysis (TEN), Stevens–Johnson/toxic epidermal necrolysis overlap syndrome (SJS/TEN)

EBC, early breast cancer

ECG, electrocardiogram

ECOG, Eastern Cooperative Oncology Group

EFS, event-free survival

EGF, epidermal growth factor

EGFR, epidermal growth factor receptor

EKG, electrocardiogram

EN, erythema nodosum

ER, estrogen receptor

ET, endocrine therapy

ErbB, derived from erythroblastic leukemia viral oncogene

FBG, fasting blood glucose

FEC, fluorouracil, epirubicin and cyclophosphamide (combination chemotherapy)

FGF, fibroblast growth factor

FGFR, fibroblast growth factor receptor

FIGO, Fédération Internationale de Gynécologie et d'Obstétrique

FISH, fluorescence in situ hybridization

FKBP12/mTOR, FK Binding Protein-12/mammalian target of rapamycin

Flt3, fms like tyrosine kinase 3

FPG, fasting plams glucose

FSH, follicle-stimulating hormone

FU, fluouracil

gBRCAm, BRCA mutated

GBS, Guillain-Barré Syndrome

G-CSF, granulocyte colony-stimulating factor

GD, gestational day

GI, gastro-intestinal

GIST, gastrointestinal stromal tumor

GFR, glomerular filtration rate

GMR, geometric mean ratio

GVHD, graft-versus-host disease

HBV, hepatitis B

HCC, hepatocellular carcinoma

HCV, hepatitis C

HER, human epidermal receptor

HER2, human epidermal growth factor receptor 2

HIV, human immune deficiency virus

HNSCC, head and neck squamous carcinoma

HR, hormone receptor

HRR, homologous recombination repair

HSCT, hematopoietic stem cell transplant

JAK, Janus kinase

KLIFS-3, kinase-ligand interaction fingerprint and structure residue-3

IAP, intra-abdominal pressure

IBC, inflammatory breast cancer

IC, immune cell

ICANS, immune effector cell–associated neurotoxicity syndrome

IFN, interferon

IL, interleukin

ILD, interstitial lung disease

ILN, interstitial lung disease

iNHL, indolent non-Hodgkin lymphoma

IRIS, immune reconstitution inflammatory syndrome

IRR, infusion-related reaction

ITAM, immunoreceptor tyrosine-based activation motif

ITP, idiopathic thrombocytopenic purpura

LBCL, large B cell lymphoma

LCIS, lobular carcinoma in situ

LFT, liver function test

LH, luteinizing hormone

LLN, lower limit of normal

LVEF, left ventricular ejection fraction

Mab, monoclonal antibody

MATE, multi-antimicrobial extrusion protein

MBC, metastatic breast cancer

MCC, Merkel cell carcinoma

mCRPC, metastatic castrate resistant prostate cancer

MEK, mitogen-activated protein kinase

MMR, mismatched repair

MRI, magnetic resonance imaging

MSI-H, microsatellite instability – high

MUGA, multigated acquisition

NCI-CTC, National Cancer Institute – Clinical Toxicity Criteria

Nib, small i**n**hi**b**itory molecule

NMIBC, non-muscle invasive bladder cancer

NRH, nodular regenerative hyperplasia (of the liver)

NSCLC, non-small cell lung cancer

OHSS, ovarian hyperstimulation syndrome

ORR, objective response rate

OS, overall survival

PARP, poly (ADP-ribose) polymerase

PCE, polymerase chain reaction

pCR, pathological complete remission

PDGF, platelet-derived growth factor

PDGFR, platelet-derived growth factor receptor

PFS, progression-free survival

Ph+, Philadelphia chromosome positive

PI3K, phosphatidylinositol 3-kinase

PI3KA, phosphatidylinositol-4,5-bisphosphate 3-kinase catalytic subunit alpha

PJIA, polyarticular juvenile idiopathic arthritis in patients aged 2 years or older

PJP, *Pneumocystis jiroveci* pneumonia

PK, pharmacokinetic analysis

PKA, protein kinase A

PMBCL, primary mediastinal B cell lymphoma

PML, progressive multifocal leukoencephalopathy

PNET, progressive neuroendocrine tumor (of the pancreas)

PR, progesterone receptor

pRb, retinoblastoma protein

PS, performance score

PsA, psoriatic arthritis

PsO, plaque psoriasis

RA, rheumatoid arthritis

RAF, rapidly accelerated fibrosarcoma

RCC, renal cell carcinoma

RECIST, response evauation criteria in solid tumors

REMS, Risk Evaluation and Mitigation Strategy

RET, "rearranged during transfection"

ROCK, Rho-associated protein kinase

ROS, 'orphan' receptor tyrosine kinase

rb, retinoblastoma (gene or protein)

r/r, relapsed/refractory

scFv, single-chain Fv fragment

SCARS, severe cutaneous adverse reactions

SCLC, small cell lung cancer

SERD, selective estrogen receptor degrader

SEGA, subependymal giant cell astrocytoma

SIRS, systemic inflammatory response syndrome

SLAM, signalling lymphocytic activation molecule family (CD319)

SJS, Stevens–Johnson syndrome

SLL, small lymphocytic lymphoma

SYK, spleen tyrosine kinase

SWFI, sterile water for injection

TALEN, transcription activator-like effector nuclease

TBC, tuberose sclerosid complex

TCH, docetaxel, carboplatin, and trastuzumab (combination chemotherapy)

TCR, T cell receptor

TEN, toxic epidermal necrolysis

TNBC, triple negative breast cancer

TMB- high, tumor mutational burden - high

TNF, tumor necrosis factor

TPS, tumor proportion score

TRK, tropomyosin receptor kinase

ts DMARD, targeted synthetic disease-modifying anti-rheumatic drug

Tyk, tyrosine-protein kinase

UC, urothelial cancer

UGT1A1, uridine diphosphate-glucuronosyl transferase 1A1

ULN, upper limit of normal

VEGF, vascular endothelial growth factor

VEGFR, vascular endothelial growth factor receptor

Made in the USA
Coppell, TX
04 November 2026

11218593R00119